PSYCHOANALYSIS, THE NHS, AND MENTAL HEALTH WORK TODAY

Psychoanalysis. the NHS, and Mental Health Work Today is one of a series of low-cost books under the title PSYCHOANALYTIC IDEAS which brings together the best of public lectures and other writings given by analysts of the British Psycho-Analytical Society on important psychoanalytic subjects.

Series Editor: James Rose

PSYCHOANALYSIS, THE NHS, AND MENTAL HEALTH WORK TODAY

edited by

Alison Vaspe

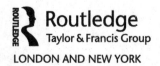

Routledge
Taylor & Francis Group

LONDON AND NEW YORK

First published 2017 by
Karnac Books Ltd.

Published 2018 by Routledge
2 Park Square, Milton Park, Abingdon, Oxon OX14 4RN
711 Third Avenue, New York, NY 10017, USA

Routledge is an imprint of the Taylor & Francis Group, an informa business

British Library Cataloguing in Publication Data

A C.I.P. for this book is available from the British Library

  ISBN 9781782203681 (pbk)

Edited, designed and produced by The Studio Publishing Services Ltd
www.publishingservicesuk.co.uk
email: studio@publishingservicesuk.co.uk

CONTENTS

v

For
Mary Banks

and for
Siobhan O'Connor
in memoriam

ACKNOWLEDGEMENTS

I owe a debt of gratitude to the many people who have helped me to think in the course of putting this book together.

Family, friends, and close colleagues have been encouraging and interested, and I want to thank them, especially Katherine Fine, who was generously and supportively alongside throughout, and Tim Dartington, who encouraged me in the book's beginnings. Dr Jacqui Ferguson, Justine Manricks, Sally Reckert, Thea de Moel, Jane Johnson, and Frangie Hutton read chapters and made perceptive and helpful comments. In addition, readers of individual chapters have made valuable suggestions, namely: Mary Banks, Andrew Cooper, Pauline Drummond, Dr Jane Garner, Dr Susie Graham-Jones, Natalie Hart, Dr James Johnston, Marilyn Miller, Kathy Nairne, Miranda Passey, Nigel Potter, Dr Mark Pietroni, Dr Patrick Pietroni, Dr Teresa Pietroni, Michele Roitt, Vega Zavier Roberts, and Dr Judith Trowell.

As series editor, Jim Rose has generated a creative spirit, as well as offering guidance from his invaluable experience of bringing books from first idea to publication.

Finally, Peter Vaspe, as well as being a valued reader, has witnessed (in the best sense of that word) the process of this project, and has borne with my preoccupation.

Julia Britton trained as a child and adolescent psychotherapist at the Tavistock Centre and worked in the NHS for many years before joining Open Door, a voluntary sector therapeutic service for adolescents and young adults in Haringey, North London. She became Director in 2013.

Tim Dartington is a writer and a group and organisational consultant, with affiliations to both the Tavistock Institute and the Tavistock & Portman NHS Foundation Trust. He has directed the experiential Leicester Conference on authority and leadership in organisations and is a member of OPUS (an Organisation for Promoting Understanding of Society) and ISPSO (the International Society for the Psychoanalytic Study of Organisations). He has a PhD for his work on developing a systems psychodynamic approach to health and social care and is the author of *Managing Vulnerability: The Underlying Dynamics of Systems of Care* (Karnac, 2010).

Clare Gerada qualified as a doctor in 1983 from University College, London. She meandered through training in medicine then psychiatry before general practice and became a partner in 1992. She has been at the same partnership since. She is now Medical Director of a sick doctor service, the Practitioner Health Programme, and was voted by *Woman's Hour* as being one of the most powerful women in the UK. She loves being a GP and especially that transitional space between doctor and patient where the magic of healing takes place. She is currently training to become a group analyst.

Richard Ingram is a consultant psychiatrist and psychoanalyst who works full time in the Belfast Health and Social Care Trust. He provides medical psychotherapy services to regional forensic and general psychotherapy services. He also has an active interest in psychoanalytic training and is Chair of the Northern Ireland Association for the Study of Psychoanalysis, a member institution of the British Psychoanalytic Council.

Amanda Keenan has worked in child and adolescent mental health services for over twenty-five years. Initially, she practised as an occupational therapist, before retraining as a child and adolescent psychotherapist at the Tavistock Centre and gaining a Doctorate in Child Psychoanalytic Psychotherapy. She is currently employed as the Lead Child and Adolescent Psychotherapist in Specialist CAMHS serving Leicester, Leicestershire, and Rutland.

Marilyn Miller is a psychoanalytical psychotherapist who trained and then taught at the Tavistock Clinic for many years. She went on to lead mental health, family, and children's services in the City of London and St Bartholomew's Hospital. Later, she developed a "body and mind" stress management package with her former partner, Patrick Pietroni, at the University of Cincinnati, which became the foundation of their interprofessional and interagency work at Marylebone Health Centre and the University of Westminster during the policy changes of the Thatcher years. She is now a Governor of the Tavistock and Portman NHS Foundation Trust and continues in private practice in Shropshire. She spends the rest of her time riding dressage and revising her play, "Ero(e)s", which explores unconscious primal scenes found in T. S. Eliot's *The Waste Land*.

Turlough Mills, MBChB, MRCPsych, PGDip, is a consultant psychiatrist specialising in child and adolescent mental health. He works with the Leeds CAMHS Outreach service and also provides Inreach psychiatry to a Young Offender's Institute and to a secure children's home. He has completed a Masters degree in the Foundations of Psychoanalytic Psychotherapy through the Tavistock and Portman Trust and is training as a Balint group facilitator. He is currently helping to develop a Leeds based service for young people with developmental trauma and associated personality development difficulties. His research interests include the phenomenology of belief systems.

Carine Minne is Consultant Psychiatrist in Forensic Psychotherapy at Broadmoor Hospital West London Mental Health Trust, and the Portman Clinic, Tavistock & Portman NHS Foundation Trust. She is also a psychoanalyst with the British Psychoanalytical Society.

Siobhan O'Connor was a psychoanalyst and consultant psychiatrist, who worked in Northern Ireland and at the South London & Maudsley NHS Foundation Trust, London. She died in 2014. Two tributes to her life and work, by her colleagues, Dr Richard Ingram and Dr Carine Minne, appear as Chapter Four of this book.

Christopher Scanlon, DPhil, has a background as a consultant psychotherapist in general adult and forensic mental health. He is a training group analyst at the Institute of Group Analysis (London), Senior Professional Associate at the Tavistock Institute for Human Relations (TIHR), and Visiting Professor, Psychosocial Practice, at the University of East London. He is a Founder member of the Association for Psychosocial Studies (APS), member of the International Society for the Psychoanalytic Study of Organisations (ISPSO) and an associate of the Organisation for Promoting of the Understanding of Society (OPUS).

Judy Shuttleworth trained as a child and adolescent psychotherapist at the Tavistock Centre. She has worked in both hospital and community settings in London and as a clinical teacher at the Tavistock Centre. She was head of child and adolescent psychotherapy in Enfield CAMHS before moving into paediatric mental health liaison at the Whittington Hospital in north London.

Wilhelm Skogstad is a psychiatrist and psychoanalyst, and a Fellow of the British Psychoanalytical Society. He works as a psychoanalyst in private practice, and is a training analyst for the British Psychotherapy Foundation and the Association of Child Psychotherapists. From 1995–2015, he was Consultant Psychiatrist in Psychotherapy and latterly Clinical Lead at the Cassel Hospital, a specialist psychotherapeutic in-patient service for severe personality disorders. He has published widely, in the UK and Germany, on issues of psychoanalytic theory and technique, in-patient psychotherapy and psychoanalytic observation of organisations. He teaches regularly in the UK and Germany and is one of the founders and organisers of the British–German Colloquium, a biannual conference of British and German analysts.

Michael Smith, MBChB, MRCPsych, MMedSci, is a consultant forensic psychiatrist. He works at Stockton Hall hospital, which is a medium secure unit in York run by Partnerships in Care. He maintains an interest in psychotherapy and undergoes personal psychotherapy.

Joanne Stubley is a consultant psychiatrist in psychotherapy and the clinical lead for the Tavistock Trauma Service. She is a member of the British Psychoanalytical Society and is also trained in trauma-focused cognitive–behavioural therapy and eye movement desensitisation and reprocessing (EMDR). She is co-Chair of the Royal College of Psychiatrists' Psychotherapy Faculty Task group on Historical Child Sexual Abuse and has a special interest in complex and developmental trauma.

Kyriakos Thomaidis-Zades is a child and adolescent psychotherapist who trained at the Tavistock Centre. He originally qualified in social work and worked in therapeutic communities for adolescents in both Greece and the UK. He currently works at the Specialist Eating Disorders Team and at the CAMHS in-patient unit in Leicestershire CAMHS.

Alison Vaspe is a psychoanalyst and psychoanalytic psychotherapist. She has worked therapeutically in the public sector for over twenty years, most recently with mental health staff experiencing psychological and emotional difficulties in the course of their work. She has written papers on the subject, and was co-author with Marilyn Pietroni (now Miller) of the book *Understanding Counselling in Primary Care: Voices from the Inner City* (Churchill Livingstone, 2000). She currently works in private practice in Hampshire.

STATEMENT OF CONFIDENTIALITY

This book refers to private and organisational issues that have been generously shared by people in the knowledge that they will not be personally attributable.

For this reason, the contributors have protected the identity of those individuals and organisations whose experiences are being described; where appropriate, the permission to publish has been sought from those whose circumstances are being specifically discussed.

This book is dedicated to two people who have made valuable contributions to mental health services. Mary Banks, who was unstinting in her commitment and care as manager of a highly effective, psychoanalytically informed counselling service for mental health staff, and Siobhan O'Connor, in memoriam, a psychiatrist who was courageous in employing her own psychoanalytic mind in order to think about very ill patients on psychiatric acute and intensive care units.

This is an important book. It concerns the contribution that psycho-analysis makes today to the provision of mental health care through the National Health Service (NHS). The book begins by looking at a number of examples of this contribution, which are written by those who are actively engaged in the delivery of these services. This gives a very direct expression of the value of applying psychoanalytic ideas to mental health care. The reader will be able to gain an insight into the experience that patients have when they are helped in this way.

These chapters also describe the experience of those who provide this kind of help to patients. They look at various settings, offering different kinds of care, and at the nature of the work that takes place in them. Thus, the reader will learn about both the experience of patients and of those whose task is to try to help them. It is in recog-nition of the fact that professionals who provide these services neces-sarily open themselves to the experience of those who suffer from mental illness. This is much easier said than done, causing consider-able stress if this is to be achieved effectively.

Therefore, to be effective, professional staff members require support to deal with the challenges and rigours of this kind of work. The second part of the book considers examples of this aspect of the provision of services, and looks at the resources required in order to create a robust setting within which appropriate service delivery can be achieved.

People seek these services because they are truly suffering in ways unimaginable to those who are not personally familiar with this kind of distress. The essential value of these descriptions of the work of providing mental health services is that they give an insight into the experience of helping these people. Psychoanalysis is primarily concerned with someone's experience and offers a conception of the workings of the mind, which has been widely appreciated and acknowledged. It has also provided the basis for the provision of services for those suffering from unbearable experiences of life for many years.

The thoughtfulness with which each contributor to this book has approached his or her subject will be apparent to all. It reflects the care and attention that they give to those who approach them for help and their capacity to respond to their problems of experience in a responsible way.

James Rose PhD
Editor of Psychoanalytic Ideas Series

Introduction

The tiger in the room: recognising the unconscious mind in mental health work

Alison Vaspe

... some day, the conscience of society will awaken and admonish it that the poor have just as much right to help for their minds as they already have to life-saving help offered by surgery; and that the neuroses threaten public health no less than tuberculosis ... When this happens, institutions or out-patient clinics will be started, so that men who would otherwise give way to drink, women who have nearly succumbed under their burden of privations, children for whom there is no choice but between running wild or neurosis, may be made capable, by analysis, of resistance and of efficient work. It may be a long time before the State comes to see these duties as urgent ... whatever form this psychotherapy for the people may take, whatever the elements out of which it is compounded, its most effective and most important ingredients will assuredly remain those borrowed from strict and untendentious psycho-analysis. (Freud, 1919a, pp. 167–168)

Freud came to England in the summer of 1938, twenty years after giving voice to this vision of a society able to be concerned with the minds of its people. As a refugee from Vienna, he had witnessed the savagery of the First World War, and then, in the 1930s, the brutalities of anti-Semitism, which, among other attacks on minority groups, found expression in the form of mob rule. His examination of the human psyche had always taken into account the destructive forces of jealousy, greed, and envy. These two world wars reinforced the need to go *Beyond the Pleasure Principle* (Freud, 1920g), giving centre stage to aggression and the death instinct as forces in their own right, rivalling the libido's drive towards life.

Although he did not live to see the founding of the NHS, or the important part played by psychoanalysis in the development of its mental health services, Freud received a warm welcome in London, where psychoanalysis was an established part of the culture of enquiry into the psychology of the mind. His arrival was considered of sufficient public significance to be reported in the *Manchester Guardian* (Gay, 1988, p. 630). Indeed, in my own family history, there is a story from the early 1940s, showing Freud's ideas to have had a currency that went well beyond psychoanalytical circles. My grandfather was a scientist and manufacturer of optical instruments who "delighted in his absent-mindedness". One evening, he left a briefcase of papers, some involving classified information, in the Underground: "They were found and returned to him in a parcel by the Air Ministry, the book he had been reading on the top—Freud on 'Forgetfulness'"[1] (Menzies, 1960, p. 275)

It is important to recognise the role of psychoanalysis in the early days of the NHS. The questions being asked in the wake of two devastating World Wars were informed by a belief in the power of the unconscious mind, and of neurosis as a determining factor in problematic and antisocial behaviour. The authors of this book ask their questions in this same psychoanalytic spirit, looking to the concepts that originated in the work of Freud, his daughter Anna Freud, Melanie Klein, W. R. Bion, Michael and Enid Balint, Tom Main, Donald Winnicott, and other psychoanalysts working in Britain before and after the Second World War, in order to address the mental health issues of today.

Mental health problems are increasingly recognised for their impact on twenty-first-century lives. Of the one in four adults in Britain who suffer from some form of mental illness, most will suffer from disorders such as depression and/or anxiety, which may be relatively mild and short-lived, but which can be severely disabling. At the other end of the spectrum are those who suffer from psychotic illness, which will prevent them from being able to live their lives in ordinary ways involving work, relationships, or enjoyable social activity. In addition, there are those who have been traumatised by their experiences of world events, such as refugees and veterans of armed conflict, and survivors of acts carried out by those whose mental disturbance leads them to behave in damaging and destructive ways. The questions asked in 1948, when the NHS was founded, remain all too relevant, as do the projects that were initiated in order to study their possible solution. However, in a political climate, which has been described as "neoliberal", it is difficult to sustain that earlier, post-war determination and sense of hope and idealism for a better future. As Bell (2013) notes,

> mentally ill people in England have been deeply affected by two main kinds of change: on the one hand, changes in the structure and scale of the health services available to them; on the other, a profound change in the cultural context in which they live . . . The rise of neoliberal values, now espoused by all the major political parties, and accelerated and intensified by "austerity", has produced a deep shift in . . . our sense of community, our obligations to and for each other . . . welfare provision is no longer seen as something that provides people with the basic necessities of life, as part of the duty of the state, but as a mechanism by which people are disempowered, creating in them a helpless state of invalidism.

This book emerged from a belief that now, as then, it is vitally important for society to understand the causes and consequences of mental ill health. Therefore, I make no apology for looking to history before turning to the contemporary context in which this book is set. In the psychoanalytic tradition, I look back, the better to go forwards.

* * *

When the NHS was founded, in 1948, there were two main strands of psychoanalytic practice in Britain. In London, Ernest Jones had been working since before the First World War to create a London-based organisation that would promote psychoanalysis. In psychiatry, the movement towards the therapeutic treatment of patients with psychological disturbance had encouraged an interest in developments on the continent: "There was a despairing need among professionals as well as patients for more therapeutic optimism, expressed in the wish, as early as 1905, to establish early treatments before asylum admission became necessary" (Hinshelwood, 1995, p. 139). With the problem of soldiers suffering from "shellshock", and unable to return to their regiments to fight, the influence of psychoanalysis on therapeutic treatment strengthened:

> Medical opinion during the [First World] war has . . . passed through three stages . . . At first treatment was largely dominated by the tradition of the Regular Army, and the usual prescription was rest, sometimes diversified by massage or electricity. In the second phase the value of suggestion became evident, the numerous disappointments following rest-cures having opened the minds of those in charge to appreciate the startling and often dramatic results of the suggestion method of treatment. Thus the way was paved for the third stage, in which it was recognised that a large number of cases treated by suggestion broke down in the firing line, or even before the firing-line was reached; it was then that the analytical method came seriously into vogue. (Crichton Miller, 1920, pp. vi–vii)

In the same year as he published this book, titled *Functional Nerve Disease*, Crichton Miller founded the Tavistock Clinic:

> one of the first out-patient clinics in Great Britain to provide systematic major psychotherapy on the basis of concepts inspired by psychoanalytic theory for out-patients suffering from psychoneurosis and allied disorders who were unable to afford private fees. (Dicks, 1970, p. 1)

However, as Crichton Miller was at pains to make clear: "The physician who has been trained to regard disease solely from the organic point of view, and the psychotherapist who has become accustomed to think exclusively in terms of mind, are both employing only monocular vision" (Crichton Miller, 1920, p. 4). The Clinic's identity as "a medical institution, not wholly committed to the then still much-feared and suspect psychoanalytic school . . . made this new approach more acceptable and 'respectable' to British medicine in the 1920s" (Dicks, 1970, p. 2).

This same approach now came to be applied to preventative and social medicine, not just at the Tavistock Clinic, which was part of the NHS from the start, but also forming part of the work of the Cassel Hospital in Richmond, Surrey, which, unlike the Tavistock, maintained an entirely psychoanalytic approach as a therapeutic community. Both organisations extended the psychoanalytic enterprise far beyond the clinical settings of psychotherapy departments, clinics, or hospitals, into the public life of a country recovering from the trauma of war, and determined to find a better way forward.

In the early 1950s, Balint began running seminars offering psychodynamic training for GPs. In 1957, Tom Main at the Cassel also began to meet with GPs, initially to think with them about the referrals they were making for in-patient psychotherapy, and then to discuss the daily problems they faced in their practices. Similar groups were set up for health visitors and probation officers. Work and school "malingering", "nerves" and neurotic unhappiness as factors in problems ranging from school failure to the breakdown of marital relations, psychosomatic illness, the prevention of potential criminality, as well as preventative work with those considered in danger of mental breakdown—in all these areas, psychoanalysis was one of the important schools of thought that were employed to bring insight to the work of psychiatrists, psychologists, educationists, general practitioners, social workers, and others involved in the prisons, schools, psychiatric, and other mental health settings that made up public life.

Separate from the Tavistock Clinic, the continuing existence of the Tavistock Institute of Human Relations allowed the receipt of research grants, which bolstered the NHS income, helping to counter the effects of the "economic stringency . . . which has never disappeared from Health Service provisions" (Dicks, 1970, p. 192). A series of systematic research studies was carried out by the Clinic from 1948–1949, when subjects included two investigations into "events in early life believed to give rise to maladjustment and psychiatric illness" (one product of this was James Robertson's classic film, *A Two-Year-Old Goes to Hospital*); an extended study of "psychoanalytic interpretation both in groups and individual therapy"; a "pilot study of methods of helping couples in marital difficulties and breakdowns"; and an enquiry into psychosomatic illness. Another important aspect of the Institute of Human Relations was the study of organisations, which had its roots in Army psychiatry, notably in the work of W. R. Bion, who sought to understand, not just neurosis in the individual, but in relation to the group to which he or she belonged, and, ultimately, to society:

Society has not yet been driven to seek treatment of its psychological disorders by psychological means because it has not achieved

sufficient insight to appreciate the nature of its distress. The organization of the training wing [of a military psychiatric hospital] had to be
such that the growth of insight should at least not be hindered. Better
still if it could be designed to throw into prominence the way in which
neurotic behaviour adds to the difficulties of the community, destroying happiness and efficiency . . . (Bion, 1961, p. 14)

[S]ociety, like the individual, may not want to deal with its distresses
by psychological means until driven to do so by a realization that
some at least of these distresses are psychological in origin. The
community represented by the training wing had to learn this fact
before the full force of its energy could be released in self-cure. What
applied to the small community of the training wing may well apply
to the community at large; and further insight may be needed before
whole-hearted backing can be obtained for those who attempt in this
way to deal with deep-seated springs of national morale. (Bion, 1961,
p. 22)

From Bion's continuation of this work, in a series of small study
groups at the Tavistock Institute, there developed a method of study-
ing the dynamics of leadership and authority within groups. This was
a precursor of the group relations approach, with which many staff
working in mental health will be familiar from attendance at events
such as the Leicester Conferences. In other areas, too, projects initiated
at this time continue to be of use. For example, "Balint goups", as well
as being important for GPs, also play a part in the training of psychiatrists (Mills & Smith, 2015). And both the Tavistock Clinic and the
Cassel Hospital remain centres of excellence for the psychoanalytic
treatment of serious psychological problems, alongside other forms of
psychological and bio-medical treatment.

In the face of the decommissioning of psychoanalytic services that
is taking place across the NHS, there is a serious movement now to
tackle the issue of outcome and evaluation, which psychoanalysis and
psychoanalytic psychotherapy have been accused of failing to
promote (Fonagy & Lemma, 2012). In the field of direct treatment, the
results of significant research projects are appearing. These include
the first randomised controlled trial in the NHS, which establishes
that long-term psychoanalytic psychotherapy provides relief for
chronic depression that has not been helped by antidepressants, short-
term courses of counselling, or cognitive–behavioural therapy
(Tavistock Depression Study: Goldberg & Taylor, 2015). Equally

important is the contribution made by those assisting mental health staff to think about the work they do—therapeutically, when the disturbance they are dealing with has an impact on them personally, or in the context of supervision, reflective practice and other groups, and organisational consultancy.

This book includes examples from all these areas of psychoanalytic work. Part I is mainly concerned with the treatment of troubled children, adolescents, and adults, as individuals and in groups, with chapters from general practice, a trauma centre, child and adolescent NHS and voluntary settings, and an in-patient hospital unit for women suffering from psychotic breakdown. Part II considers the impact on staff, and the challenges to organisations and their managers, of working in mental health. Chapters explore the contribution made by consultant psychiatrists and reflective practice groups to mental health teams, the value of incorporating a "participant–observer" approach into a senior clinical management role, the therapeutic treatment of mental health staff who themselves experience psychological difficulties in the course of their work, an exploration by an organisational consultant on why it is important that those who manage mental health services care for those who are doing the caring, and an interview with Dr Clare Gerada, MBE, a leading figure in the field of general practice, followed by an analytic commentary in a postmodern context, on the relationship between the "self and the system" in the GP setting.

To some extent, the two sections overlap. Accounts of psychoanalytic treatments refer to the need for psychoanalytic models of consultancy and other forums for therapists to reflect on the work they do. Addressing the need for staff to have time to reflect on their experiences at work, in order to reduce burn-out, sickness absence, and early retirement, and the effects of developing a "thick skin" (at worst leading to abuse of vulnerable patients), is also viewed as a vital factor in providing more effective care for patients, and as generating new ideas about why recovery may not be forthcoming.

One corollary of this is the book's use of the term "patient", rather than client or service user, for all those whose "suffering" (Latin *patientem*: "bearing, supporting, suffering, enduring") is being held in mind, whether they are recipients of mental health services, or providers of them, in the knowledge that working in such settings is, by its nature, psychologically challenging, and often disturbing.

As in the early days of the NHS, mental health work is viewed in its wider, socio-political context. There is recognition of the relevance of social conditions for understanding psychological suffering. Psychiatric institutions are no longer viewed as "bins", in which these problems can be disposed of: these authors write from an understanding of the ways in which individual neuroses and psychiatric disorders reflect the psychological problems of wider society, where, as Bion says, they destroy both "happiness and efficiency".

* * *

In Chapter One, a central psychoanalytic concept is defined in the context of the general practice setting. Marilyn Miller's examination of the different ways in which a multi-professional team employed the term "containment" revealed its "transformative" potency, but also found it was used to describe ways of working with patients that could be defined as of a "safety-net", or "repressive", kind. The team found it painful to recognise the ways in which they could gloss over the gap between a wish always to work in ways that transform patients' lives, and the reality: "that only about one third of the activities in general practice are transformative, one third are to do with sustaining the *status quo* and preventing deterioration, and one third are to do with managing an individual or family situation which is deteriorating and will go on doing so whatever interventions are made". The work put in achieved an important, shared recognition of the institutional task, and an awareness of the social defences that all the practitioners came to realise they were using, in order not to suffer the anxiety of knowing their limitations in the face of patients' suffering.

These three definitions have a useful, broad application to the book as a whole. Some of the chapters focus on contributions to mental health work that can be described as "transformative", while others aid understanding of the strain for staff of "practising disappointment" (Scanlon: Chapter Eight). All mental staff have to bear the reality that "cure" may not be possible, but that patients may benefit from help in managing their lives in better ways, or where containment of a "repressive" kind is necessary, because their vulnerability puts them or those around them at risk of injury or death if they are not restrained, medically or physically.

Chapter Two examines another psychoanalytic concept, which is closely linked to containment. From her work with patients suffering the consequences of developmental trauma, such as childhood sexual or physical abuse, or adult trauma, as refugees, war veterans, victims of torture or domestic violence, and political incarceration, Jo Stubley looks back to Freud's attempt to understand trauma among soldiers serving in the First World War. Hearing of their repetitive nightmares prompted him to review his idea of the dream as a product of wish fulfilment, and to formulate the concept of a death instinct, which pushes against the efforts of the life instinct. Stubley shows how she employs countertransference—initially viewed by Freud as problematic, given the analyst's need to be neutral in the face of the analysand's difficulties and distress—in order to understand the emotional experience of her patients. This understanding helps these patients to form their own psychological narrative, and, hence, develop a sense of self-mastery. Stubley is aware, as she works in the confidential and intimate relationship allowed by the clinic setting, of other professionals around the patients she works with: the nurses, housing workers, doctors, and psychiatric staff, whose efforts might be met with psychic collapse, self-sabotage, or negative emotional responses, when relief and hope might have been expected.

Another important development originating in the work of the Tavistock Clinic was the use of observational studies, both as a means of understanding organisational functioning, and also in the study of early mother–infant relationships. In Chapter Three, Judy Shuttleworth and her fellow authors explore the contribution of psychoanalytic thinking about children and adolescents to their work as psychotherapists in the NHS and in voluntary settings. They place observational studies at the centre of their understanding, employing case vignettes to show the importance of noticing behaviours, such as missed appointments and late arrivals. With the help of experienced psychotherapists, the meaning of such behaviour can be understood, not as indicating poor motivation, but as complex communications, which, translated into words, can help these young people to think about their experiences and the choices they make in their lives.

The chapter is imbued with the importance of history—both for the young people in need of insightful attention and for the services themselves, which, despite the numerous ways in which psychoanalytic psychotherapy has contributed to the delivery of child and adolescent treatment, are at risk of being overlooked. In addition to providing in-depth treatment, the application of psychoanalytic understanding was applied to the development of brief therapy, to the forming of a team response, or to helpful discussion, which contributed to the understanding of other professionals working with young people, using different techniques. However, as the authors note, this success was double-edged:

> these clinical developments were not characterised in a way that emphasised their difference from what went before [and so] with the arrival of evidence based practice [and] a new generation of evidence-based "brand name" treatments and related trainings . . . [i]t has been much harder for those treatments, such as psychoanalytic psychother-apy, that emerged out of clinical practice prior to this change to develop a research methodology appropriate to the nature of the treat-ment and to gain the funding needed for an evidence base.

The consequences are not just of concern to the child and adoles-cent profession. The authors suggest that the nature of clinical prac-tice itself is in danger of adapting to the needs of the research base, rather than to the needs of the children and young people who most need help. At worst, a "technical", symptom-based, problem-solving approach might lead to those with more serious needs being consid-ered ineligible for treatment. Failed by the system, they are likely to feel that it is they who have failed to meet its requirements for illnesses that conform to existing research methodologies.

In Chapter Five, following two tributes, by Richard Ingram and Carine Minne (Chapter Four), we remember the work of the late Siobhan O'Connor, to whom this book is dedicated. Her in-depth study of aggression on an all-female psychiatric intensive care unit (PICU) emphasises the skill and depth of thinking required in mental health work. Originally written in the context of a commitment to banish mixed-sex wards in NHS Trusts (Department of Health, 2002), O'Connor's chapter is also relevant in the light of a more recent "shared commitment" by the previous Conservative–Liberal Democrat Coalition Government and leading health and social care organisations (DoH, 2013) to "end the institutional divide between physical and mental health, primary and secondary care, and health and social care".

O'Connor observed how a medical model of illness took priority in the minds of doctors and nurses working with the very vulnerable women on her ward. At the same time, she found herself affected by what seemed an inability of the staff on this ward to think. She recognised the impossibility of meeting patients' needs in an effective way if every in-patient bed was filled, all the time: "If one cannot focus upon the complex medical problems, the risks are high, and that was my main concern when I asked for a reduction in beds for a period". Applying her psychoanalytic mind to the dynamics on the ward, she observes the importance of continuity of care for women when psychotic states are likely to reflect difficulties in relating on a pre-oedipal level, which might be quite inaccessible unless a sensitive and sustained alliance is made. Furthermore, while acknowledging the importance of excluding organic illness as a contributory factor in psychotic states, she also warns of the need for physical interventions, which may need to be intrusive, to be carried out within a therapeutic alliance, in order not to create further disturbance in the patient. She considered that the exposure of repeated transfers in specialised services might have exacerbated the illness in those for whom a therapeutic relationship was an equally essential aspect of their treatment.

All these chapters, which have the primary aim of exploring the role of psychoanalysis in mental health treatment, make reference to the importance of psychoanalytically informed consultancy, supervision, and groupwork for staff, in order to aid understanding of the needs of patients, and also of the impact of the work on the individual. In Part II: "Organisational and staff needs and challenges", each chapter explores the difficulties presented to mental health staff and organisations as they attempt to respond to the concrete and anti-thinking tendencies of those in their care. The *Francis Report* (2013) is in the minds of all these authors, who work as clinical leads, as clinical and organisational consultants, in reflective practice and other groups, and therapeutically, when staff themselves become unwell. There are commentaries on the pressures of inspection, which might be experienced as undermining of clinicians, and on the "skewed" nature of evaluation (mentioned by Shuttleworth et al. in Chapter Three), when it is made to serve information technology, rather than being served by the undoubted advantages and advances of our modern capacity to collect data. Thought is given to the self-awareness required if, for example, Care Quality Commission inspections or audit and evaluation are to result in a true reflection of the clinical needs of patients, rather than straying into the seductive terrain of "virtual reality" (Hoggett, 2010). The complexity of organisational life in the NHS is viewed from the perspective of the GP, who stands at the front-line of most initial mental health presentations, and needs to navigate the system on the three levels of what Miller (Chapter Eleven) calls "the ABC of organisational life".

In Chapter Six, two consultant psychiatrists show how they employ psychoanalytic thinking in their work with children and adolescents in the NHS, and with adults in forensic secure services in the private sector. As part of their specialist and sub-specialist training, they studied psychoanalysis and undertook the work of being patients in psychoanalytic psychotherapy themselves. They note the essential importance of accepting the limitations of knowing—a stance that may be at odds with other models of mental functioning used within psychiatry—using case illustrations to show that being able to bear "not knowing" is important if staff are to resist an impulse to act in order to discharge disturbing feelings in damaging ways.

A more integrated view of psychiatric medicine, in which "the psychodynamic psychotherapeutic viewpoint was [propounded as] the cornerstone of all psychiatrists' skills" (Dicks, 1970, p. 285), was supported by the incorporation of Balint groups into the training of psychiatrists in the 1960s—and in the area where Mills and Smith both work, as a form of reflective practice group for higher level trainees also. The value of such groups, in their capacity to hold and contain the powerful anxieties and emotions that emerge in the course of mental health work, is further explored by Chris Scanlon in Chapter Seven: "Working with dilemmas and dis-appointments in difficult places: towards a psycho-social model for team-focused reflective practice".

Scanlon's concern is for the damage that can result if staff's experiences are left unattended. In the context of staff health and wellbeing, there are consequences that must be borne by the organisation if mental health workers are allowed to become burnt-out and ill. But also, in our post *Francis Report* era, following the scandal surrounding abuse of vulnerable residents and patients, including and especially the elderly and those with severe learning disabilities, we know all too well that staff can behave in "monstrous" ways.

Outlining the training, skills, and experience required to facilitate such groups to best effect, Scanlon notes the need for management to take responsibility for the reflective practice project in order for there to be a "feedback loop" connecting the anxieties held at this senior level with the clinical anxieties of the staff.

In Chapter Eight, Wilhelm Skogstad writes of the high level of self-awareness that goes into his own senior role as Clinical Lead of an in-patient unit at the Cassel Hospital, and of how this underpins the success of the treatment provided to patients suffering from severe personality disorders. With its focus on communality, aimed at promoting the social capacity to care for self and others, the treatment is intensive, operating on the level of the individual and the small and large group, paying attention to the different activities and dynamics of day to day living, as well as to specialised analytic work. This awareness extends beyond the patient groups and their relations to staff, to thinking about staff relationships and dynamics, the culture of the organisation, how this influences the beliefs and assumptions of those within it, to complex management and NHS policy concerns, and the dynamics surrounding them.

Skogstad provides a case example of his own responses while heading up a treatment unit where powerful and disturbing anxieties were aroused by working with a vulnerable patient group, with tendencies to self-harm and suicide. He shows how unsettling pressures come from all directions—the inevitable comings and goings among staff and patients, the impact of external demands for audit and inspection, visits by the Care Quality Commission, enquiries following untoward incidents, and spending reviews. Only by maintaining a steady analytic attention was he helped to resist the pressure to act, or react.

Skogstad's stance as an observing participant helps him to recognise the pressures that senior NHS managers and policymakers are under, and the ways in which he, too, feels caught in a culture of blame, which can seriously undermine clinical care. At its most extreme, the clinical manager can lose sight of real concerns affecting patients and staff, becoming caught up in a kind of virtual reality, where boxes ticked and targets met can provide a veneer, concealing the complex demands of the work with patients and the needs of staff for containment.

In Chapter Nine, I consider the contribution of an in-house, psychoanalytically orientated staff counselling service, and the ways in which broad concerns can be fed back to the organisation, without breaching confidentiality, in order to help senior managers think about difficult staffing issues. The chapter centres on an individual case study, involving a mental health nurse from an in-patient, older

xxxiv   INTRODUCTION: THE TIGER IN THE ROOM

adults unit, who was the subject of an enquiry into circumstances surrounding a patient's death. The chapter explores the motivation of staff who feel impelled to "blow the whistle" on the workplace, the vulnerability of those who enter into the vocational work of caring, for deeply personal reasons, and the need for careful thought to be given to their likely responses to distressing situations, including their own life experiences, which may have an impact on issues they are dealing with at work. Citing some commentaries on the *Francis Report*, which singles out the elderly as needing specialised training, the chapter supports recommendations for there to be more attention to the needs of staff, not just for training and skills, but for encouragement in thinking about their own feelings surrounding old age and death.

In Chapter Ten, Tim Dartington explores the dynamics of care "to see how it may be difficult at times for those whose business is managing therapeutic interventions to show compassion towards those who are doing the work". His concern is that containment of staff has become a "neglected management function"; the consequence is a system that lacks the capacity to be self-reflective, which is essential for compassionate care. Working from his professional role as an organisational consultant, he explores the anxieties inherent in the work of care and our complex and conflicted response to need. If our anxiety about vulnerability, which exposes us to fears of being in danger, is not contained, the system that is supposed to support compassionate care becomes a receptacle for our own unwanted projections of inadequacy into others. He reminds us of the crucial importance of all the spaces available to staff, which allow them to reflect on their work, including: "the most informal, at the water fountain or the canteen, or the pub when someone is leaving, or those structured occasions, coaching and non-managerial supervision and reflective practice groups, counselling, away days, CQC inspections". All these meeting points provide ways to acknowledge the unconscious and subconscious emotions—"of love and hate"—as well as the anxiety and potential sadism that we may experience when faced by the vulnerability of others.

Chapter Eleven returns to the general practice setting, with a dialogue between Marilyn Miller, a psychoanalytic psychotherapist with experience both of senior management and of governorship in an NHS mental health Foundation Trust, and Dr Clare Gerada, MBE, who was Chair of the Royal College of General Practitioners (RCGP) between 2010 and 2013. Starting with Gerada's account of her personal journey, as a GP's daughter, they make a detailed exploration of how relentless changes, over many years, affect GPs' ability to do their work. Chapter Twelve provides a companion piece to this, in the form of Miller's analytic commentary, describing the postmodern context within which general practitioners work—a complex organisational system of assessment and referral—and the unconscious factors evoked by the doctor–patient relationship.

In her ABC model of the system, Miller shows the three different levels GPs have to navigate. Within this, the GP must "find a way, every ten minutes, within a crowded morning surgery, to match diagnostic 'rigour' with a 'relevant' (and rapid) response that fits the needs of the patient, any relevant guidelines, and the constraints, where applicable, of local contracts agreed by CCGs".

The scene Miller and Gerada describe is shown, beneath the apparent order of regulated computer systems and work processes, to be chaotic, beset by constant policy changes, and demands always to do "more for less". Methods of mass production, the supermarket, SatNav type directives and protocols, and the discontinuity of care when GPs are expected to hot-desk and work with patients like cab drivers on Uber taxi ranks, rather than develop a relationship with their own patient list as the family doctor once did—these are the ways of working that seem closest to a "new NHS business culture [that] is tearing apart GPs, and other workers within it".

This chapter brings to a close a series of accounts showing some of the many and various contributions currently made by psychoanalytic practitioners to working with the troubling aspects of our minds, which find their most acute and chronic expression in the field of mental health.

In my "Concluding remarks", I return to the central focus of this book: the need for psychoanalytic thinking to be available to staff, in different ways, in order to help them sustain the difficulty of their work. I look to the larger problems facing us today—in particular the damage we are causing the environment—and borrow the description of a form of mental ill-health adumbrated by the psychoanalyst Sally Weintrobe, in her book on climate change (2012). We live, she suggests, in a "culture of uncare", characterised by defences based on omnipotence and denial. I end, considering what our contemporary equivalent might be of Freud's compassionate vision of mental health treatment made available to the minds of all those who need it. Can we draw upon the psychoanalytic understanding developed within our NHS mental health services to benefit wider society? Can we develop Bion's suggestion that at least some of society's distresses and difficulties are psychological in origin and offer "whole-hearted backing . . . for those who attempt in this way to deal with deep-seated springs of national morale"? (Bion, 1961, p. 22).

* * *

These authors show us how analytic understanding can be applied in primary, secondary, and tertiary settings, both to create brief models of therapy with individuals and groups, children, adolescents, adults, the elderly, and to mental health staff themselves, and to inform the ordinary practice of mental health staff, through clinical consultation, supervisory and reflective practice work in groups and teams, and in the consultancy provided to senior managers and to organisations.

However, the chapters also offer a commentary on a contemporary scene, in which NHS services are struggling to provide an adequate level of care to mental health patients. There is frequently a sense of crisis narrowly averted, and of staff brought close to breakdown. These commentaries raise serious concerns about resources and staffing levels; about a culture that can seem to condemn and exclude the vulnerable, rather than seek an empathic understanding of them; and about ways of measuring care that give a "virtual" picture, remote from the reality of patients' experience.

In this "target culture", performance and box-ticking might be privileged over care of the person, and staff are subjected both to over-scrutiny of tasks reduced to "aliquots" of care and to continuous and destabilising change. The reality of good pockets of thoughtful, effective work, with a wholehearted engagement from staff wanting to make a difference to people's health, both mental and physical, must be seen in this context, which has been described by the neurosurgeon and author Henry Marsh in troubling terms: "The subtle balance between vocation and money at the heart of healthcare has been entirely destroyed" (*Guardian* Opinion, 27 April 2016). Good, vocational healthcare staff are treated as though they are "just another group of assembly-line workers" and "medicine as just another business" (Marsh, 2016).

Of course it is true, as Miller reminds us (Chapter Twelve), that in some ways it is a good thing for practitioners to be held to account. The question is whether this is done in a punitive way, or in a spirit of enquiry. It is very difficult, in the former case, for a healthy, necessary professional defence to be employed in the service of reflection and informed decision-making. In its place can come a professional defensiveness, with managers feeling wrong-footed, caught between patient distress and the political wish to be seen to be getting it right.

There is a growing body of work that addresses these concerns. Organisations such as the Point of Care Foundation, the Royal College of Psychiatrists (Johnston, 2017), and the General Medical Council are calling for change including the need for psychoanalytic thinking and reflective practice to be returned to mental health work. There are studies that focus on the need for care to be informed by "intelligent kindness" (Ballatt & Campling, 2011). Important psychoanalytic texts go further, addressing the powerful anxieties operating in the work of physical and mental health (Hinshelwood & Skogstad, 2000; Menzies Lyth, 1988a[1959a]; Obholzer & Roberts, 1994) and the problematic effects of a "primitive mind of state" (Bell, 1996), the imposition of a bullying, "target culture" (Evans, 2014; Francis, 2013; White, 2013), and the ways in which our public health services can operate in fragmented and isolated ways that resemble pathological, "borderline" functioning (Cooper & Lousada, 2005). By developing our understanding beyond the simplistic labelling of individuals as evil or, as good nurses are often described, as "angels", institutional abuse can be recognised as a systemic issue, reflecting political problems at the highest level. More, it is stated, is required than the sacking and prosecution of individual culprits, who may be sent as scapegoats into the wilderness, in the hope that they will take with them the serious problems that bedevil our public institutions.

Given the scale of the problem, it may be argued that making a case for psychoanalytic thinking in what is left of the NHS is missing the larger point, of resources and business practice within what is becoming a care "industry". However, the truth is that most of our understanding of the mind, developed over nearly seventy years, since the founding of the NHS, was and is inspired and informed by psychoanalysis, and that this body of knowledge is woefully underemployed. We could do so much better, and we need to, because mental health matters.

As those employed in the early days of the Tavistock Clinic were aware, it matters that we understand the conditions that promote a productive and motivated society. Such an understanding is all too often a casualty of the delegation of care to a privatised, market system, following the passing of the Health and Social Care Act (2012). This Act has replaced a professionally led health service, directly accountable to the Secretary of State for Health, with a competitive tendering culture, in which accountability and responsibility for the commissioning and providing of NHS services are the remit of an NHS Commissioning Board and a plethora of independent, local, Clinical Commissioning Groups. Many of those involved with the NHS are deeply concerned about its capacity to survive in a form that can come close to the best of what has previously been available: good healthcare based on clinical need, available at the point of delivery, regardless of wealth or ability to pay.

In her book, *Tigers in Red Weather*, the poet Ruth Padel wrote about her journey to those parts of the world where tigers can still be found, asking why it matters that the wilderness should continue and wild tigers exist. Perhaps her description of the eco-system in which tigers can be found offers a way to think about how we can provide mental health settings that foster awareness of the presence of unconscious forces that affect our ability to think in creative and constructive ways. She writes of the relationship between the wild animal and the land-scape for which it evolved—the way in which

> Tigers need prey, water, cover. If they have all they need, everything else in the forest is all right too . . . Everything depends on everything else: the tiger is top of all. If you save tigers, you save the whole thing. (Padel, 2005, p. 25).

To have the skill and ability to catch sight of the unconscious mind at work could be considered akin to seeing a tiger in the wild—a sign that the system, in which mental health problems are supposed to be treated and understood, is supporting staff in the careful monitoring of their own minds, in order to find some insight into their patients' disturbance and distress. The eco-system in which they are enabled to do this involves a safe and secure environment, a well-functioning, well-managed system, adequate and appropriate staffing, good com-munication between teams and organisations, continuity of care,

adequate, skilled supervision, and other formal and informal opportunities to think with colleagues. Mental health work does not rely on
expensive equipment to be effective. It relies on good minds and good
hearts, and the conditions that allow these to develop.

The chapters in this book represent the benefits that accrue when
psychoanalytic thinkers and clinicians have these opportunities. The
authors have given generously to showing how they face the challenges of working in mental health today, using their capacity for care
to find ways to counter the negative forces that also exist in human
nature, and which are in danger of running wild, if not checked by the
containment of public services that represent the constructive efforts
of society at its best.

Or perhaps another way of saying this is that it is safer to see the
tiger—to know the dangerous and destructive, as well as life-giving
capacities we are all capable of having—than to turn our back on it out
of fear, and pretend it does not exist.

PART I

PSYCHOANALYTIC APPROACHES
TO WORKING WITH PATIENTS

CHAPTER ONE

Theory in use: perspectives on containment*

Marilyn Miller

From high ground to swamp

I begin the chapter with a brief exploration of the psychodynamic meaning of containment, which, though complex, has been opened up by some useful commentaries (Hinshelwood, 1989; Meltzer, 1978; Moustaki, 1981; Symington & Symington, 1996). Those with a psychodynamic orientation will be familiar with the origins and meaning of the term, which has frequently been applied to the worlds of counselling, psychotherapy, and family therapy, following its development in the psychoanalytic world in the 1950s (e.g., Box et al., 1981; Wiener & Sher, 1998). I hope that other members of the primary health care team less familiar, or enamoured with, the psychodynamic literature will find this bird's eye view of the concept useful, not least because the argument will move from the psycho-analytic origins of the term to its varied use in the more eclectic culture of the multi-professional team.

---

* This chapter was originally published as part of a book on counselling in general practice (Pietroni & Vaspe, 2000). It is reprinted with some revisions by kind permission of the publishers, Elsevier Ltd.

A link is made between the original specialist definition of containment, usually attributed to Bion (1959), and the development of the idea of the "flash" technique in the work of Enid and Michael Balint, which is very familiar to most general practitioners. Like Bion, both were psychoanalysts, and their concept of something communicated in a brief general practice consultation in a disorganised way suddenly becoming crystallised, understood, and available for examination has some common features with Bion's concept of containment, where something communicated unconsciously, and often beyond words, emerges into consciousness (Balint & Norell, 1973).

I then move on, in Schön's terms (1987), from this theoretical high ground to what he called the swamp of everyday practice; by examining the range of rather different meanings in use for the term containment, discovered in two years of multi-professional debate in the monthly Marylebone Health Centre academic meetings. This part of the chapter shows how a sophisticated concept developed in a specialist setting can be, and has been, adapted to a generalist one, where a range of different philosophical, theoretical, and clinical models necessarily co-exist. This adaptation is not seen as a form of "dumbing down". Rather, an examination of the different meanings in use is seen as an important reflective exercise if a multi-professional team is to develop the capacity to work inter-professionally with the kinds of problems that are thrown up by life in a capital city. Too often, such a team can hide behind different professional languages in which the same word is used without awareness that it means something quite different to different members and has quite difficult practical implications. It would have been easier, for example, to concentrate only on the psychotherapeutic use of the term without reference to the contradictory uses in the team as a whole. Instead, we start with our own perspective and then trace it through the somewhat unsettling multi-professional debate and surprising discoveries that were made in the academic meetings.

Containment of the psyche–soma: the psychoanalytic origins of the term

Containment is not an easy concept to understand or to put into practice. However, thanks to the work of Hinshelwood (1989), it is now possible to identify the origins of selected psychoanalytic concepts fairly easily. He has done a wonderful job of defining concepts and mapping the development of their different meanings across a range of primary and secondary sources. Hinshelwood describes containment as a "decisive concept" and points out its close links to Melanie Klein's concept of projective identification "in which one person in some sense contains a part of another" (p. 246). He chooses a quotation from Rosenfeld to show the developing relationship between these two terms, a quotation which is illuminating from the point of view of general practice because it refers implicitly to physical as well as mental experience, and it is often the body that patients first bring to the GP as the container of the symptom of their inner dis-ease.

> The patient . . . showed that he had projected his *damaged* self containing the *destroyed* world, not only *into* all the other patients, but into me, and had changed me in this way. But instead of becoming relieved by this projection he became more anxious, because he was afraid of what I was *putting back into him*, whereupon his introspective processes became severely disturbed. (Rosenfeld, 1952, pp. 80–81, quoted in Hinshelwood, 1989, p. 244; my emphasis)

The words "damaged", "destroyed", "into", and "putting back into him" convey a physicality behind their abstraction that allows one to imagine, in a kind of shadow-play alongside the adult verbal exchanges, the mime-like movements of a child's sometimes violent interaction with another. What the quotation makes clear is that containment is a powerfully felt, active, and interactive process, which involves a process of shredding and projecting what are felt to be damaged, frightening, or unwanted parts of the self for psychosomatic containment inside another.

Freud had written many years previously that the ego that mediates between different levels of consciousness (within and between individuals) is, in the first instance, a body ego: "The ego is ultimately derived from bodily sensations, chiefly from those springing from the surface of the body" (Freud, 1923b, p. 26). He explained the relationship between sense perceptions, which have their origins in the body (hearing, sight, touch, taste, smell), mental images (which he considered to be primitive: "Thinking in pictures is . . . only a very incomplete form of thought", 1923b, p. 21), and words.

Thus, he laid the ground for Bion's work on container–contained, which discriminates between communication where emotional life and depth can be tolerated, however confused, violent, or inarticulate, and communication, which is hollow or emotionally empty, or uses dissociated physical signs, where the emotional links between thoughts, words, and psyche–soma have been unconsciously severed. Hinshelwood summarises Bion's view of these vital links as follows: "Thus putting experiences into thoughts and thoughts into words, entails a repeated chain of linking processes modelled on physical intercourse between two bodily parts" (Hinshelwood, 1989, p. 341).

The container–contained relationship

Bion defines containment in terms of a shifting container–contained relationship (1962). The concept is based on the model of the mother as a container for the infant's projected needs, feelings, and unwanted parts. A defining feature of what has to be contained is that either it has not reached a verbal state, or it has burst open the capacity of words to contain meaning. Bion gives the example of the stammer, where emotion disrupts the containing forms of words and grammar. The containing other receives this pre-verbal raw material and is then involved in a reflective psychosomatic process in which psychic diges-tion takes place alongside disciplined physical awareness. Therefore, the process of understanding what is being contained requires emotional labour of a profound psychosomatic kind and is not simply sitting and listening, important though that is.

The concept of containment, or the container–contained relation-ship depends heavily on two other linked concepts, which are techni-cal and also somewhat difficult to understand: projective and introjective identification (Klein, 1946). Rosenfeld's quotation, cited above, shows these interactive processes of identification at work. The patient tries to get rid of some unwanted, uncomfortable, damaged part of himself by projecting it into another (or others) using the mech-anism of projective identification. The psychosomatic stuff projected by the patient for containment into the inner space of the containing other is often somatically felt before it is psychically recognised. Indeed, it might not actually be psychically recognised and might remain pre-conscious for some time. Either way, the process of containing such inchoate, primitive material is referred to as introjec-tive identification. Something has been overtly or covertly pushed into the container, who now carries and is changed by it. The container's powers of observation, reflection, and discriminating, though, determine to what extent the projected and unwanted part of the self can later become consciously articulated and reintegrated.

Containing can, therefore, be likened to a process of psychic digestion, in which the container's senses first receive and examine (chew over) what has been projected before the next stage can begin: the emotional and cognitive work of separating what was felt to be mental poison or waste matter from what is psychologically useful and needs to be reintegrated by the originator. Then a new stage of "making sense", or articulating, what was previously inchoate can begin. The containment process is somewhat paradoxical: precise and disciplined on the one hand, chaotic and confusing on the other.

Bion uses the term reverie to describe the calm and receptive state of mind required of the containing other who is ready to introject and make sense of what has been projected (1962). The container, in a state of reverie, identifies at a primitive psychosomatic level with the "undifferentiated stuff" that has been taken in and only then begins to sift and try to understand it, before going on to detoxify the more alarming aspects and eventually finding a safe enough means of expression. This process eventually allows the modified contents to be returned in a safer and more tolerable form.

The model provided by the container of not only surviving the process of containing such hazardous material, but also being able to distil and return it as something useful, offers a model of the container–contained relationship that can itself be introjected. In the future, a reservoir of repeated experiences of self-containment strengthens inner resources sufficiently for them to be drawn on repeatedly, even under duress. The active container–contained relation provides a model for continuing personal development.

The prototypical psychosomatic origins of the model are described by Bion as the mother and infant, or, more primitively, the nipple and breast, penis and vagina, and it is to these prototypes that Hinshelwood is referring when he uses the term "physical intercourse", as quoted above. This movement in description in the literature between body metaphors and mind metaphors reflects the complexity not only of the concept of containment and therefore the relation between container and contained, but also of the living relation between body and mind, a relation which is central to the task of understanding that faces practitioners with each new patient, especially in the general practice setting, where patients usually present with a physical sign in the first instance. When a patient such as a "Torture victim" (Pietroni & Vaspe, 2000, Chapter Ten) is referred to the counselling service, or a "Refugee artist" (Chapter Eight) who is struggling for mental life in the face of heavy anti-psychotic medication, or an "Uprooted schoolgirl" (Chapter Eleven), caught between languages, it is not unusual for the main means of communication to be through projective identification, with little use of words. The quality of containment provided by the counsellor is then vital to the patient's mental survival and development.

Containment in the general practice setting: links with Balint's "flash" technique

The concept of containment reviewed above derives originally from the theory and practice of psychoanalysis. As a concept related to practice technique, it is usually familiar to therapists and others trained psychodynamically. Although GPs train differently, they have their own historical links with psychoanalytic thinking, some of which might be unfamiliar to psychodynamic therapists. As one might expect, the rather different terms used reflect the economy of response expected of a GP in a brief consultation, but, on closer examination, the ideas have much in common.

The nature of the GP–patient consultation was looked at in depth, drawing on a psychoanalytic perspective, by Michael and Enid Balint (Balint, 1964; Balint & Norell, 1973). For many years, GPs met in "Balint seminars" at the Tavistock Clinic and elsewhere, presenting their cases for discussion with a psychoanalyst or psychoanalytical psychotherapist to examine in depth the unconscious aspects of the doctor/patient relationship.

Balint drew on this work when he described the "flash" technique, which, though quite different in some respects from Bion's concept of containment, is similar in others, especially in terms of the quality of listening required (Bion's reverie) and its paradoxical combination of freedom and discipline. The "flash" technique moves away from the traditional aim of "pinpointing the seat of the trouble" to an alternative aim of "providing the patient with the opportunity to communicate whatever it is s/he wants" in a "brief, intense and close contact" and following up on what has been communicated in such a way that a shared moment of understanding occurs that allows what follows to have an emotionally substantial quality, sometimes with and sometimes without practical implications.

Enid Balint, describing how to develop the liberation of the "flash" technique, described three working principles:

1.   The doctor should not be *too* preoccupied with theories or preconceived questions.
2.   The doctor needs to consider what to do with his/her observations.
3.   The doctor needs to respect the patient's right to hide or not disclose his/her secrets.

In her development of these principles, the links between the "flash" technique (familiar to GPs) and the use of containment (usually familiar to therapists) becomes more evident. Both depend on that quality of listening, described by Bion as reverie, that allows clarification of meaning to emerge from both unconscious and conscious sources, and is often registered psychosomatically. Enid Balint's chapter "The 'flash technique': its freedom and its discipline" (Balint, 1973) suggests further links between these two important concepts (see Figure 1.1).

If one has a theory, one is limited by the theory; if one has not theory, it is difficult to observe . . . but it gives freedom to observe. This freedom is only useful if it is coupled with discipline: in our case the discipline of careful and attentive observations, and the ability to know how much of what is observed originated with the patient and how much is contributed by the doctor him/herself . . .

The difficulty is more in keeping up the intensity of attentive observation after a decision has been made to comment or interpret . . . The doctor has to reflect silently about his observations and their meaning: identify with the patient, develop ideas about him, and then to intervene by making a comment or interpretation to test out his line of thought. As we know, the silent reflecting part of the process is done very rapidly.

Figure 1.1. The Balints' "flash" technique: links with Bion's containment (from Balint & Norell, 1973, p. 20).

Implications for practice

Awareness of social defences

If a practitioner can use these abstract ideas about how to listen and how to think about what a patient is communicating, it does not necessarily mean that s/he "gets it right". Nevertheless, it does help the work in an important way. Smith (1992) writes of "the emotional labour" required of professionals if they are to combat the worst forms of stress arising from their work in ways that do not involve building up a thick defensive skin.

Often, professionals build up a defence against the repeated pain, frustration, helplessness, and intimacy that confronts them in their work as a way of surviving, and this is encouraged in basic training as part of establishing the appropriate distance of a boundaried professional identity. GPs, psychological therapists, nurses, and complementary therapists, for example, engage with the most private aspects of either the bodies or the minds of their patients and sometimes both. They and their patients need help in managing this intimacy from a mutually understood repertoire of role behaviours, which involve different kinds of distance regulation.

Professional distance is necessary but it can be overdone. It can become a kind of protective habit worn to convey confidence and purity, to conceal uncertainty, to impart a false sense of expert knowledge, or, most important of all, to establish and sustain membership of a professional tribe with its hierarchical internal class system. Here, Schön's distinction between the "expert practitioner", who assumes expert knowledge and establishes distance from the client, and the "reflective practitioner", who recognises the limits of professional knowledge and establishes a sense of partnership and connection with the client in a joint exploration, is relevant.

The attempt to contain a range of often disturbing psychosomatic communications in a brief period of time, therefore, involves a tension between the distance required to allow productive reflection to occur, and the intimacy needed to be available and useful as a container. Menzies Lyth's classic article (1988b[1959b]) describes the social defence systems used by a nursing hierarchy in a teaching hospital. She shows only too clearly what happens if the anxiety about letting something disturbing in is allowed to generate a defensive social system based primarily on distance: staff morale drops, sickness rates increase, and attention is displaced on to organisational rituals, which are of minor importance, while the real nursing tasks are neglected. So, too, it can be in general practice, whether one is a doctor, nurse, counsellor, receptionist, or complementary therapist. A defensive "thick skin" can be created that inhibits the capacity of the individual professional to think independently and to use initiative and imagination. The thick skin also ensures that the patient's communications bounce off, rather than being taken in, thought about, and responded to appropriately.

When, in the next section, we turn from theory to practice, it becomes clearer just how such social defences find expression and how contested the idea of containment really is. When the members of a multi-professional general practice team were given the space to struggle openly with the meaning of the term containment (and, therefore, with this tension between distance and intimacy), they discovered they were using it in different and contradictory ways.

Containment of the psyche-soma: an exploration of the meanings-in-use in the multi-professional team

When Marylebone Health Centre staff spent six of their monthly academic meetings examining what was meant by the much used term containment when used by different members of the multi-professional team, it became clear that there were almost as many meanings in use as there were members in the team.

The counsellors used the term in much the way outlined above, as originally defined by Bion, meaning that some kind of useful transformation was felt to be possible if a difficult (confused, painful, violent, inarticulate) communication could be taken in, "chewed over", detoxified, and handed back in a recognisable and more bearable form, making it available internally for future use.

The GPs used the term containment frequently, but rarely meant the same as the counsellors. More often, they meant they could do little for a patient with either medical treatment or advice, so what was possible was simply to provide some kind of support or safety-net.

When the complementary practitioners used the term, they tended to mean something similar to the GPs. Occasionally, however, GPs and complementary practitioners would mean something different again by the term, more akin to control or repression, for example when a patient was seriously problematic and in frequent contact with the practice in a rather demanding and difficult way that took resources from more needy patients.

The discovery of this range of three different meanings-in-use for the term containment (transformative, safety net, and repressive) led to a decision to use one year of the lunchtime academic meetings (about eight hours after holidays) looking at examples of use by the multi-professional team and generating some differentiated but shared meanings in the language of everyday speech that we could all understand and use. The choice of a shared common language was important because each profession had its own jargon or technical language that seemed to obscure differences in meaning and to impede inter-professional communication in the team.

The first year's cycle of academic meetings was an example of reflection on action; in Schön's (1983) terms, the first cycle allows change and reframing to occur within a single, relatively simple system by reflection on, or after practice. The second cycle of reflection he called "reflection-in-action", which is more complex. First, it takes place in the midst of practice pressures and not with hindsight; second, it needs to combine intuition, intellect, and professional judgement in some kind of on-the-spot experiment or improvisation, which goes against the grain of well-worn ritual and modifies basic assumptions, the apparent "givens" of everyday practice and organisational life.

A second year of academic meetings was, therefore, later devoted to applying and testing the new shared meanings on further practice examples in each of the different professional units (see Chapter Seven). This decision allowed the second cycle of reflection-in-action to occur, and provided the opportunity for promoting real organisational learning (Argyle & Schön, 1978).

Figure 1.2 contains the three definitions that were agreed at the end of this work. This is followed by a brief explanation of how the team found they were using these definitions after a further year's work.

Transformative containment

This meaning is the most complex and was used by all members of the multi-professional team but perhaps most commonly by the counsellors. As described above, it has been substantially theorised by Bion

1. *Transformative:* This patient seems to want to understand their symptoms/difficulties/behaviour and to grow/change their lifestyle/behaviour; furthermore, we think that with our help they can do so, at least to some extent. Therefore, we will take in their communication in some depth, try to understand it, and perhaps begin to help to articulate it. In the process, we will take some of the sting out of the needs and communication they are bringing to us, so that it feels safer to take them back in a newly integrated way.

2. *Safety net:* We probably cannot help this patient to become much healthier, or to learn or to grow, but we can help him/her or his/her situation not to deteriorate by being available, listening, and offering treatment, support, advice, or clarification when needed. The problem is that the patient is motivated, but for a variety of reasons (the state of our skills and knowledge, the nature of the illness or behaviour, or a lack of resources), we can help only a little and mainly in a supportive way.

3. *Repressive:* This patient seems constantly to be seeking help, often across a range of services in and outside of the practice, and often in a way that eventually wastes resources and upsets staff. By the nature of their difficulties, there is very little that we can do to help, but we need to limit the wastage of resources and the damaging impact that the patient's behaviour is having on staff. Understanding or intervening does not seem to help; the pattern of contact just endlessly repeats itself, so we have to take firm control.

Figure 1.2.   The meanings in use of containment at Marylebone Health Centre.

(1962). After discussion, the descriptive term "transformative" was selected because all professions in the team could identify with the word and the idea, notwithstanding their different world views and theoretical orientations. The meaning was finally re-stated as in Figure 1.2.

The most common use of this meaning of the term was with those patients where the GPs or complementary therapists could make a relatively quick assessment, perhaps drawing on Balint's "flash" technique, followed by some useful therapeutic intervention, or where the counsellors had a patient referred with whom they could do some constructive brief work that was likely to achieve some form of limited transformation.

Safety net containment

The most common use of this meaning of the term was in relation to long-term, seriously ill patients with severe or chronic physical illness such as heart disease, cancer, or multiple sclerosis, or with severe mental or neurological illness such as schizophrenia, dementia, severe and recurrent depression, or bipolar affective disorder. From the restated meaning, it was clear that some elements of Bion's definition of the term remained. There is a recognition that a particular quality of listening and thinking makes an important contribution to the continuing care of the patient, even if it cannot contribute in a curative way. There is also the recognition that the resource framework of the NHS cannot stretch to provide as much of this type of containment as the patient might feel is wanted or needed or the worker may wish to provide.

Repressive containment

This meaning was the most contentious. All professions recognised that there were times when they had to set exceptional limits on their interactions with patients in a way that could feel almost brutal. On the one hand, they recognised that this was part of being a professional, maintaining appropriate distance and being clear about what was and was not possible; on the other hand, there was a quality about this form of containment that made them feel uncomfortable, frustrated, and often guilty, no matter how much they tried to understand the process at work. In part, this was the effect of the patient powerfully transferring his sense of responsibility for himself on to the practitioner concerned, sometimes with the covert blessing of another member of the team. Often, this would happen between the GPs and the massage therapists to whom patients might be referred when the GP needed a break from the pressure. Usually, however, this form of containment was used because the professional (or the practice as a whole) had been "run dry" by a patient who seemed unable to take anything in but repeatedly came back for more like an insatiable baby.

In conclusion

The gap between theory and practice identified by Schön was rediscovered at Marylebone Health Centre as a result of this exercise. The team discussions were carried out in the reflective practice tradition and brought many shocks, some of them painful to us, but achieved the following important outcomes:

- multi-professional or parallel working changed to inter-professional collaboration based on a deeper understanding of difference and explicit commonalities;
- professional jargon was reduced so that more accurate communication between professionals could occur;
- social defences were identified and some of their harmful effects on the professionals and their practice were reduced (less professional isolation, reduced guilt, improved team support, clearer limits, more thoughtful responses to patients' needs, fewer "heartsink" patients created by professionals being unable to say no);
- a shared recognition of the institutional task of inner city general practice with its finite resources was established; idealism, guilt, and cynicism gave way to a greater realism.

Each different type of containment defined has a place in the services which inner city general practice can provide. Our aspiration is naturally to offer as much of the transformative approach as possible, while the reality is that only about one third of the activities in general practice are transformative, one third are to do with sustaining the *status quo* and preventing deterioration, and one third are to do with managing an individual or family situation which is deteriorating and will go on doing so whatever interventions are made.

CHAPTER TWO

Countertransference experiences as an aid to staff working with traumatised patients

Joanne Stubley

The *English Oxford Dictionary* definitions given for trauma include: "A deeply distressing or disturbing experience; emotional shock following a stressful event or a physical injury; a physical injury" (Soanes, 1998).

Of Greek origin, the literal translation is to wound. Considering these definitions, it is immediately apparent that trauma in the context of the day-to-day work of the helping professions is ubiquitous. In physical medicine, many patients will feel traumatised by the experience of both their illness and its treatment. For instance, recent studies suggest a high incidence of post-trauma symptoms in people who have received treatment in intensive care units (Johns Hopkins Newsroom, 2013). In social care, one encounters victims of child abuse or domestic violence as part of everyday work. In GP surgeries and community settings, veterans, asylum seekers, and refugees may all bring with them their particular experiences of trauma. In mental health, trauma might be part of what has led to the difficulties or might be a consequence of the experience of being mentally ill—street homelessness, psychiatric detention under the Mental Health Act, traumatic loss of jobs and families, are all potentially traumatic experiences. It follows that working with people across these different settings will inevitably face the staff with difficult experiences of their own to contend with. What I hope to convey in this chapter is a way of attempting to think about these experiences, to use them to understand our patients and clients better, and to engage in working with them in a manner that is thoughtful and humane.

I shall use a psychoanalytic understanding of the impact of trauma to describe how staff members are inevitably pulled into particular kinds of action: repetitions of the traumatic experiences that are revived at an unconscious level. If one is alert to this in the work, it may be possible to prevent situations where, although help is available, it cannot be helpfully used; instead, it becomes a kind of enclave or excursion where nothing changes. In the worst case scenario, time, effort, and money are diverted into endless cycles of unconscious repetition of the traumatic experience between patient and staff.

From a psychoanalytic perspective, trauma is thought to pierce the protective shield around the mind so that it is flooded with an excess of external stimulation. Internally, there is a powerful reactivation of primitive anxieties that further overwhelm the individual. Helplessness, chaos, and horror contribute to the sense that one's worst nightmares have been realised. Trauma attacks the capacity to symbolise, so that thought is no longer possible, at least in the area of the trauma itself. There is inevitably a push to action and one form this might take is through the power of the repetition compulsion. Traumatised patients may unconsciously construct a theatre in which the traumatic scenario is endlessly repeated, with the different roles of victim, perpetrator, witness, and rescuer offered to others who may be drawn in. Staff will find themselves repeatedly and unconsciously drawn into re-enactments of this traumatic scenario in its various forms.

The diagnosis of post-traumatic stress disorder (PTSD) has been in common usage since the mid-1980s, originally coined in response to the experiences of Vietnam veterans in the USA. Of course, trauma responses after war experiences have been known about for much longer in the psychiatric literature and have included such terms as railroad spine, shell shock, traumatic neurosis, and so on. The symptoms of PTSD include intrusive symptoms of nightmares, flashbacks, intrusive thoughts and images, and triggers for these symptoms, including intense physiological distress, avoidance and numbing symptoms, which include avoidance of anything associated with the event alongside an emotional blunting and shutting down, and hyper-arousal symptoms with hyper-vigilance and exaggerated startle response.

PTSD diagnoses include natural and man-made disasters, victims of violence including sexual violence, victims of incarceration and torture, and other events where extreme terror, helplessness, or threat to life was experienced.

In 1992, Judith Herman, an American psychiatrist, described a particular group of trauma survivors as having a condition she called complex trauma (Herman, 1992). This group included veterans, victims of domestic violence, and adults who had been sexually abused as children. She felt the link with these groups was the experience of captivity and the result was a constellation of symptoms. These included the classic PTSD features alongside dissociation, somatisation, re-victimisation, identity disturbance, and affect dysregulation. This diagnosis is not yet in any formal psychiatric classificatory system but it is increasingly recognised by clinicians as a helpful description of patients who have suffered repeated, sustained, or chronic traumatisation.

Complex trauma presentations can be found in many different clinical settings, including general psychiatry, psychology departments, IAPT services, primary care, psychotherapy departments, and specialised trauma services. Different treatment approaches and modalities may be used in working with these patients, who might have experienced developmental trauma such as childhood sexual or physical abuse, or adult trauma including many refugee experiences, war veterans, victims of domestic violence, political incarceration, and so on.

A common thread in all these settings and presentations is that the staff will inevitably find themselves faced with difficult and, at times, overwhelming emotional responses to their patients. A psychoanalytic understanding of trauma can help one to understand the impact of this work on staff and provide a space in which thought might help to intervene in the inevitable push towards action.

Case history: physical injury leading to PTSD

Mr R was referred to the Tavistock Trauma Service after sustaining serious, life-threatening injuries in a motorbike accident. He was having nightmares of the event, intrusive thoughts and images of the scene would frequently occur, he was avoiding driving a car, and felt unable to return to work. He had recently broken up with his fiancée and was increasingly isolated and depressed.

This young man in his early twenties had been successful in business in a somewhat reckless manner. He had spent much of his youth seeking out a variety of death-defying activities, including bungee-jumping, parachuting, and motorcycle racing. After the accident, Mr R seemed to have managed the months of hospitalisation and physical recovery by becoming the model patient. All of the nurses spoke of what an impressive young man he was, always doing what he should and obliging the staff in any way he could. It was after being discharged for three months that Mr R began to feel increasingly depressed, hopeless, and despairing, with the symptoms I have described.

When he came to see me, I was immediately struck by what a likeable, helpful, and obliging chap he was. However, in telling his story to me, Mr R would suddenly say something in his descriptions that had a shocking and almost jaw-dropping effect. For instance, he was speaking in a rather general way about the injuries he had sustained and then suddenly switched into giving me a minutely detailed, grisly, and gory account of exactly what his badly damaged leg had looked like at the scene of the accident. The effect on me was to feel shocked, horrified, and taken aback. When this happened again, in a slightly different context, I became more aware of a way of operating that Mr R employed. When he delivered these blows, I was momentarily left reeling and he, in contrast, seemed almost bright and breezy.

As Mr R's history gradually unfolded, he gave a vivid account of a violent, unpredictable father and a rather masochistic, self-effacing mother. Mr R remembered that as a child he would be peacefully sleeping in his bed when his father would come to him and slap him repeatedly across the face. No explanation was ever given and Mr R's mother never intervened. His response was to try to be as well behaved as possible, keeping himself hidden from his father's eyes by becoming like his self-effacing mother. My sense was that Mr R's experience of these parents, with father's unpredictable violence and mother's masochism, provided a template for his interpretation of the accident. Mr R experienced the event as a kind of unexpected, violent slap in the face. His response was to do as he had done before, become the good little boy, doing everything he was meant to in order to prevent further punishment. However, he was left with serious disability and perhaps this served to act as a kind of on-going slap, one that his usual defences just could not help him to escape from.

Freud tells us, in 1909b (p. 122): "A thing which has not been understood inevitably reappears; like an unlaid ghost, it cannot rest until the mystery has been solved and the spell broken".

For Mr R, the "unlaid ghost" of his early traumatic experiences with his father reappeared when he experienced the trauma in his adult life. It became the template for the adult trauma, giving unconscious meaning to the event that then enabled him to use similar defensive strategies to manage the anxieties that had been evoked.

One might also see how Mr R's early experiences had been given potential for re-enactment prior to the accident, for instance in his seeking out of death-defying activities. In *Inhibitions, Symptoms and Anxieties* (1926d), Freud emphasised that central to the traumatic experience is helplessness. He linked this to traumatic moments in development when one is faced with the possible loss of what is felt to be vital—loss of the loved object, loss of the object's love, loss of self-love, and so on. The unbearable nature of helplessness pushes for action, and one form of action is through the repetition compulsion. Through repetition of a traumatic experience, one can choose, at an unconscious level, to identify with different aspects of the traumatic scenario: as victim, perpetrator, witness, rescuer. Identification with the aggressor holds the promise of mastery over helplessness, activity over passivity. For Mr R to place himself in potentially life-threatening situations—albeit in a controlled manner—one can see how something frightening, threatening, and terrifying could happen in a way that was, at least in large measure, under his control. He was the one potentially administering the slap in the face to himself each time he took part in an extreme sport. However, the phrase "death-defying" is also important, as these were activities in which he defied the threat, he was the master, and prevented the slap.

When Freud described the repetition compulsion in *Beyond the Pleasure Principle* (1920g), he began with the question of why traumatised veterans presented with nightmares that endlessly repeated their traumatic experiences. This did not fit with his notion of dreams as wish-fulfilments and, thus, was not explainable through his theory of the dominance of the pleasure principle. In trying to understand nightmares as a common symptom of traumatic stress, Freud was gradually led to posit a notion of a death instinct in us all—a powerful force which ultimately pushes every organism to return to the inanimate state. From the beginning of life, he suggests, there is a powerful struggle between the life instincts and the death instinct. The repetition compulsion, while clearly representing this inevitable return to an earlier state, also holds an admixture of life and death forces, with the life instincts representing the potential for mastery, for defiance, for a new opportunity to arise.

In the room with me, Mr R invited me into the position of victim. I received the slap in the face, unexpected and unasked for, while he was identified with his father's role. Understanding this over time allowed for the possibility of stepping outside our limited roles within the traumatic scenario to begin to think about what had happened in his life—how his more recent traumatic experience had been given unconscious meaning through his childhood experiences and how this contributed to his difficulty in moving forwards after the event.

Case history: a refugee in a battle for housing

Mr A came to the UK as an unaccompanied minor after losing all his family in his war-torn homeland. He was clearly a survivor, someone who had found capacities inside that allowed him to keep going. When I met him, he had been in the country for four years and in that time he had been granted status and had successfully applied for British citizenship. He had learnt English and had begun a college course. What was occupying his mind at this time was his battle to obtain council housing. He had been made homeless after breaking his arm and losing his temporary job. He now lived in a hostel and was desperate to obtain a place of his own.

The battle with the council over the appropriate banding of his housing needs became the central preoccupation for the next two years. Over this time, I saw Mr A on a fortnightly basis and would write supportive letters when this seemed necessary. He rarely spoke of anything to do with his life prior to arriving in the UK, and I had little sense of what had happened to him until his arrival in London. Most of our time he was focused on the council and the fight he faced.

When Mr A obtained his council flat, my sense was that something inside of him collapsed. He moved into an empty, almost uninhabitable flat and broke down.

This description of the fight followed by the collapse when the aim is reached is not uncommon. As long as there is a clear fight to be won, almost unlimited internal strength might be found. The battle serves a number of purposes. First, it keeps one busy, so that the mourning that is required for the many losses the traumatised patient faces can, for a time, be warded off. Second, it allows the management of anxieties through defence processes such as splitting and projective identification. There is, of course, also the reality that these are battles that need to be fought in many circumstances.

In the Tavistock Trauma Service, we make use of Melanie Klein's description of the early infantile state of mind to understand the nature of the anxieties the traumatised patient faces and the defences at their disposal (Klein, 1946). Thus, the trauma results in a reactivation of powerful, infantile anxieties from the paranoid–schizoid position of early infantile life. The patient is overwhelmed by primitive terror and dread; anxieties of disintegration and death predominate. Terrible, frightening forces prevail and there is no sense of protection or trust in the goodness of the world. The worst of infantile and childhood fears are realised.

In the normal course of development, the way an infant attempts to manage unbearable anxieties such as annihilation and disintegration is to split their feelings and experiences into categories of very good and very bad. This helps to make the feelings more manageable; it is only slowly, as the mind develops, that it can begin to integrate its view of the world. The other defence mechanism that holds sway in these early times is projective identification. What this essentially means is that what is unbearable is split off and evacuated into the mind of another. This has an impact on the other.

In time, it might be possible to bring together these categories of very good and very bad in a way that allows for recognition of the way they are being attributed to individuals who are experienced as gratifying the patient's needs, or frustrating them. This recognition opens the possibility of more mature states of mind, involving ambivalence, mourning for what has been lost, and the recognition of one's own aggression. Guilt and the potential for reparation result, in what Klein (1940) described as the depressive position. We would see this gradual shift as a time in which development and change are possible, but at the cost of considerable psychic pain.

For Mr A, the fight with the council set up a very potent split, where the council became the bad guys and I was the good guy. In work with asylum seekers, one can often see this kind of splitting, with the resulting idealisation and denigration of the Home Office. The split allowed Mr A to manage his anxieties and to keep at bay the unbearable feelings he had in relation to his experiences. When he no longer had this split available, everything flooded back.

My experience with Mr A was to feel invited into being the rescuer. I would protect him from the terrible housing department, who were persecuting him. Of course, one of the dangers of being idealised while another is denigrated is that these positions can easily switch and this often meant I was anxious and uncertain. This was added to by my impression that Mr A was, at times, being aggressive and threatening to the housing staff, giving them an experience of helplessness and fear. His experiences of such profound trauma at a young age were literally unthinkable and, hence, he acted them out in his battles to find himself a home. One also imagines that finally winning the battle for a home overwhelmed him with guilt for being the sole survivor of his family and gaining what they had all lost.

Massive psychic trauma collapses the distinction between the external world and internal experience: there is no longer an outside from which a perception came or an inside which can register it. When the external world becomes a direct reflection of our worst nightmares, most terrifying thoughts, feelings, and fantasies, then reality testing is irrelevant and the survivor enters the world of psychic equivalence. "Psychic equivalence" was a term used by Peter Fonagy to describe how mental contents can appear to correspond to physical realities (Fonagy & Target, 1996). However, in trauma this is reversed: it is not that perception has been contaminated by unconscious fantasies but, rather, that the psyche is overwhelmed by external horrors that find their equivalents in the unconscious. Our worst nightmares are realised; thought and actuality have become one. Reflection is foreclosed and thinking and perception are replaced by concrete mental entities that cannot be explored. Bion, describing his own experiences in the trenches, emphasised how effective it can be to destroy links between thoughts during the trauma itself.

Destroying links between thoughts allows one to fend off annihilation anxiety that is proving literally unthinkable (Bion, 1959).

This has interesting connections with neuropsychological research in trauma that demonstrates the brain's failure to formulate thoughts efficiently under extreme stress.

As Van der Kolk (2014) describes, a traumatic event does not get processed in symbolic/linguistic forms, as most memories do: instead, it tends to be organised on a sensorimotor level, as horrific images, visceral sensations, or fight/flight reactions. Storage on a sensorimotor level and not in words is supposed to explain why this type of material does not undergo the usual transforming process into autobiographical narrative memory. This leads to Van der Kolk's oft-repeated phrase, that in trauma "the body knows the score".

The increased secretion of adrenaline in trauma disrupts the hippocampus, short-circuiting the system so that memories become stored as somatic sensations and visual images in the amygdala. The higher cortical structures for linguistic memory are bypassed. Fragmented sensory, affective, and motor memories bombard the survivor, often seemingly without triggers. This bombardment, coupled with the sense of being unable or unwilling to find the thoughts that might attach to them, leads survivors to be increasingly withdrawn and reactive. One can also see how this connects with presentations of medically unexplained symptoms—somatisation—a common feature in complex trauma patients.

Case history: psychiatric detention
as a repetition in complex trauma

For Ms B, her body kept the score of her prolonged torture and rape. This had occurred while she was a married woman with two children living in her war-torn homeland. She had been accused of subversive activities by the government, was arrested and imprisoned. She was repeatedly tortured and raped. In between these events she was left in a cell with one other woman, who died after several days from her injuries. Ms B was sure that she would also be killed. After several months, she was freed. Her husband was now missing, presumed dead. Ms B managed to escape across the border with her children and, against considerable adversity, found a new life for herself.

However, Ms B was plagued by headaches and chest pains, which had no known organic cause. Subsequently, she was also found to have type 2 diabetes, which was chronically poorly controlled and led to many physical symptoms. Ms B had symptoms of depression and classical PTSD features, including intrusive phenomena such as nightmares and flashbacks alongside hyper-vigilance. She was referred by the GP after she had been detained on section in a psychiatric unit for several weeks. This seemed to have arisen out of increasing concern about her mental state and she had expressed suicidal thoughts. Her GP's concern was that she was expressing her suicidality through her poor diabetic control.

The experience in the room with Ms B when I met her was to feel very rapidly tired, as I strained to listen to her high-pitched whisper. Any movement or noise would cause her to jump and scan the room for threat. I found myself frequently experiencing headaches after our meetings, accompanied by a tension, a sense of needing to do something quickly. It was rapidly clear how much anxiety Ms B had injected into the system in a manner that culminated in her psychiatric detention. She concretely experienced this as a repetition of her previous incarceration. There was an enormous push for me to become the good object who was going to protect her from these experiences occurring again.

Ms B would sit with me, holding her head, whispering her complaints against the psychiatric team, jumping if I moved or began to say anything. I found myself immobilised, helpless in the face of her distress. It was when she began to tell me the story of the other woman in her cell that it was slowly possible to see how much her own experience of helplessness was being enacted. As we began to consider this together, it also became possible to think about her fury and how much of this was being directed against her own body. Ms B's interaction with health and social care professionals seemed to invite a small number of possible responses, which I slowly became aware of, in the transference relationship with me. Thus, one was encouraged to be the good object, the rescuer who would protect her from harm. Otherwise, the push was towards action, which Ms B then experienced as persecution and torture, repetitions of her previous traumatic experience. Or one was left helpless, in the manner I have described.

My sense was that Ms B had been unable to symbolise what had happened in her traumatic experiences, and, thus, mourning was impeded. The guilt, fury, pain, and sadness were avoided and, instead, action ensued in the form of various identifications within the original traumatic scenario. It was as though her body had become both the prison that held her and the helpless, suffering object of torture. Ms B was using her body to act out a masochistic state of mind that used suffering as a means to avoid persecutory guilt, and this could be traced in the transference relationship with me and in what had been acted out with her psychiatric admission. The physical symptoms represented a kind of refuge from something dangerous and persecutory internally that needed to be contained.

What is interesting about Ms B's experience is that at different times she enacted different aspects of the trauma: identification with the aggressor, which I experienced in the transference, feeling helpless and pinned down by her anxiety and with her treatment of her own body, identification with the dead or damaged object in her melancholia, and identification with the victim state in her interaction with the psychiatric team and the repetition of her incarceration through the hospitalisation.

In the work with Ms B, the initial phase of establishing a therapeutic alliance focused on the need to contain the considerable impetus for action. This was evident in the wider system in terms of her recent sectioning and in the transference. Trauma may be viewed as a failure of containment whereby the overwhelming of existing structures and defences against anxiety attacks the links between self and other. The repetition compulsion pushes for what cannot be thought about to be repeated instead, over and over again. Thus, Ms B plays out the drama of her traumatic experiences in each new encounter, including in the room with me and in an ongoing way in her body.

In describing something of my emotional response to being with Ms B, I am giving a description of my countertransference experience. Countertransference—the feelings aroused in the analyst—was initially seen as an obstacle to therapy, as was transference itself. A more modern view of both is usefully captured in Joseph's (1985) description:

> [the transference] . . . must include everything the patient brings into the relationship. What he brings in can best be gauged by our focusing our attention on what is going on within the relationship, how he is using the analyst, alongside and beyond what he is saying. Much of our understanding of the transference comes through our

understanding of how our patients act on us to feel things for many varied reasons; how they try to draw us into their defensive systems; how they unconsciously act out with us in the transference, trying to get us to act out with them; how they convey aspects of their inner world built up from infancy—elaborated in childhood, experiences often beyond the use of words, which we can often only capture through the feelings aroused in us, through our counter-transference, used in the broad sense of the word. (p. 447)

Traumatised patients have been overwhelmed with primitive anxieties, which they defend against by using primitive defences of splitting, projection, and projective identification. The use of projective identification, as described by Klein, is an unconscious phantasy in which the patient expels contents, usually of a disturbing kind, into the other. This influences both the analyst's state of mind and her affects, and might have an impact on her behaviour, in what are called "enactments". Through enactments it is possible to know about unconscious identifications and primitive modes of functioning in a way that would not otherwise be possible.

In working with traumatised patients, aspects of the relationship that emerge in the room between patient and therapist are a reflection of the early experiences that have been taken by the mind to provide meaning for the traumatic event. Use of the transference relationship through close monitoring of one's countertransference experiences enables a deeper and more thorough exploration and understanding of the meaning of the traumatic event for that patient. Discovering the unconscious meaning of the event allows the patient to make sense of the way they have responded to the traumatic event, but also how they are continuing to play this out in their current relationships, including enactments within the therapy and encounters with other professionals.

Case history: a traumatised refugee

Ms C suffered significant injuries when she was the victim of a suicide bomber in a United Nations building in her Middle Eastern homeland. She was a Christian who was brought to the UK for medical treatment and subsequently applied for asylum. In the midst of all this, one of her brothers was kidnapped and tortured. When I met her, she spoke of her hatred of this country and her mistreatment here. She was often disturbingly racist and attacking of Arab people and felt threatened by Muslims. When Ms C spoke of the English with hatred and disdain, or of the Home Office and its treatment of her, I would find myself thinking, "Well, thank goodness I am Australian, so she can't mean me."

My sense is Ms C was desperately trying to find a way to keep her original home safe in her mind and that this required splitting off anything dangerous or bad into others who were different. Davids (2011) writes of this in his paper on the internal racist, describing the capacity in us all to lodge what is unacceptable into the other, who is recognised as "not like us". I believe my sidestepping of this process, in my thoughts of my own identity, was an attempt to avoid the painful reality of what Ms C was attempting to manage, which included her own aggression and fury with the English, who made her feel so vulnerable, needy, and dependent. It is often true that these feelings of dependency are heightened by the system of asylum, where one is unable to work, often dependent on the charity of others, and passively required to await outcomes of proceedings that could take many years.

Working with Ms C was often a very painful and difficult experience. She would speak very rapidly and in a loud, shrill voice that would feel at times as though it was reverberating inside my mind, leaving me with a headache. (It is interesting to note that her major symptom after the bomb was severe headaches.) When she would utter racist comments in this manner, it was often difficult to feel that I could think sufficiently to address this in a robust way. I would find instead that I was left uncomfortable with having somehow gone along with her racism. The experience for me in the room was repeatedly to find myself anxious, guilty, and unable to think.

My sense is that Ms C was communicating something she found disturbing and unbearable, through projective identification. Trying myself to bear her communication, without action or attempts to rid myself of the pain and acute discomfort, was essential to my beginning to offer her an emotional experience, which, psychoanalytically, Bion (1959) conceptualised as containment. Bion described this notion in terms of the experience mothers offer their babies. In the normal course of development, a baby, filled with the kinds of early anxieties I described earlier, communicates this distress emotionally. It is the mother's role to try to take this in, to think about it, and attempt to understand what might be going on in the baby's mind so that she might relieve this distress. Over time, with repeated experiences of containment, the baby builds up a reliable experience that someone can bear what they feel is unbearable. This can lessen the baby's need simply to be rid of distress, and instead help him or her to find ways to think about such experiences.

Ms C had every reason to feel herself in the grip of terror, dread, and anxiety that was both annihilatory and persecutory. She was trying to manage by splitting her experiences and her feelings so the new country became the bad guy and the old held everything good. She attempted to rid herself of what was unbearable through her racism. Her communication with me was a powerful experience, where I was being asked to contain something of what she could not bear. The containment in this way is also something that I feel is part of providing a home—hopefully a temporary one—for what cannot yet be borne. In time, Ms C has slowly been able to move more towards her ambivalence for both countries and has no longer spoken of racist feelings. It has been possible to mourn some of what she has lost and to feel more curious about her new country.

Case history: historical child sexual abuse

Ms X is a thirty-year-old African woman, who was referred by a social worker after she instituted criminal proceedings against her former foster carer. The court case was now pending. The referrer felt Ms X needed neutral ground to allow her some support in this period of her life.

There was something rather split and incongruous in Ms X's narrative as it gradually presented in the consultation. Her initial appearance was of a competent young woman, who I learnt had recently finished a degree. She appeared thoughtful, available to interpretations, and aware of her emotional difficulties. And yet . . . I found myself thrown at the start of each consultation session by the almost complete change in her appearance: hairstyle, clothes, and accessories—all were re-done to present a dramatically different image. In a similar vein, I would suddenly find myself startled by a piece of material that felt psychiatrically psychotic. For instance, she suddenly began to tell me how a popular singer had stolen all of her poems from the internet and used them in her lyrics.

The attempts to understand Ms X's narrative—the question of what had happened to her—was a frustrating and seemingly impossible task. Gaps, discrepancies, and inconsistencies were rife in her story and left one feeling uncertain of anything. Ms X had, it seemed, been sent from Africa to the UK at the age of four. She was placed in foster care, alone and unprotected in the face of chronic sexual and physical abuse by at least three people, including the foster mother. At sixteen, she was given a flat on her own by social services. Her history was scattered with repeated episodes of abusive relationships with men, drug and alcohol abuse, eating disorder symptoms, impulsivity, and affective instability. Five years ago she had been raped and was made homeless. She was now in stable accommodation, had her degree, and was working part-time.

In the work with Ms X, I continued to have the sense of not knowing who would come into the room. I struggled with a countertransference feeling of wanting to know, to address the ambiguities and uncertainties in her history. I began to see how this linked with a pull into being potentially intrusive with questioning, or else feeling neglectful and uninterested if I did not act in this way. I would find that if I made interpretations, these would often seem to be taken at a very concrete level. Her responses would leave me uncertain whether she was talking metaphorically or was actually psychotic. Time and thought in the trauma unit with my colleagues allowed some sense of needing to hold this uncertainty. As a group, we thought it suggested a way in which she was also profoundly uncertain of me, and of what kind of object she was with. It would feel as though she simply did not know how to differentiate good from bad. This was played out during this time in a relationship she began with a married man, which certainly had an element of sadomasochistic interaction, but which she would bring as though it were something good and supportive. Food would, at times, have a similar quality, where she would move between bingeing and starving, with an uncertainty whether this was something dangerous or essential to life. I would often feel very anxious about her suicide potential and the degree of social isolation that appeared to surround her.

Hume and Kleeberg (2004) write of a similar experience in working with a group of people who had been abused in an orphanage as children, and who were now being offered therapy funded by social services as the police investigation prepared to take the perpetrators to court. Their experience in this setting was captured in the idea of "corruption" in the countertransference. The therapist experiences a confusion and uncertainty in the work, linked with the patient's confusion between good and bad. Early experiences of abuse by carers might lead to an internal world where objects may well be perverse, neglectful, often crazy, but almost always mixed, so, at the same time, experienced as loving and needed. It is this confusion that is traumatic. As they describe, "What gets established in the mind is a terrifying muddle of good and bad, of affection and hatred, so that everything is contaminated" (p. 77).

I found myself beginning to get a glimpse of something in Ms X's early experience with her mother that felt full of disturbance and neglect. It also became clear that one of Ms X's anxieties about therapy was that she would need to go back into and re-live her childhood abuse. Again, the concrete nature of this is something I took up with Ms X as an expectation of intrusion and sadism from me. Ms X also spoke of an idea that she needed to pinpoint the traumatic experience in order to move away from it. This highlights the kind of temporal relationship that the trauma paradigm can perpetuate, where the notion of retrospectively prescribing causality to events can give an illusion of certainty. For Ms X, some of the struggle, it seemed, was to allow there to be uncertainty. This need might be a reflection of much earlier disturbance. Words often seemed to represent the trauma paradox for Ms X— being simultaneously powerful and overwhelming and, at the same time, feeling puny and fragile in the face of the push for action.

Discussion

In these brief vignettes, I hope I have given some sense of the struggles that might face professionals in working with traumatised individuals. I have described my own experiences in a specialist trauma service, but I believe they are applicable across a broad range of settings and modalities of therapy. In every relationship between a professional and an individual suffering the aftermath of trauma, there are these possibilities of enactments, of repetitions of the original traumatic scenario.

What I find I, as a therapist, need to face in my own countertransference experiences can feel unbearable and there is, at times, the wish to turn away. At other times, I feel the pull to be active, to become caught up in the political and social realities of the patients' experiences, and there can be a real threat of becoming the rescuer and turning a blind eye to their resilience and capacities. Acknowledging the extent of human aggression and destructiveness that is part of the response to traumatic events is vital, when one can be unconsciously drawn into the role of aggressor or perpetrator. Careful monitoring of the countertransference experiences, often requiring support of a team or supervision, allows for the recognition of the complexity of these encounters. Ultimately, it might offer the possibility of action making way for thought, remembering rather than repetition.

Acknowledgements

I would like to thank the members of the Tavistock Trauma Service for the solid containment of working together over many years.

Confidentiality and consent

The case histories presented are a composite of cases seen over many years in the Tavistock Trauma Service and, as such, do not represent any one person's experience.

CHAPTER THREE

Thinking psychoanalytically about mental health services for children, adolescents, and their parents

Judy Shuttleworth, Julia Britton, Amanda Keenan, and Kyriakos Thomaidis-Zades

Introduction

T he aim of this chapter is to trace the contribution of psycho-analytic thinking in relation to the long development of mental health services for children and adolescents, and to place this alongside more recently emerging clinical and managerial approaches to mental health and, most recently, the national reorganisation of these services that is now under way. We describe, first, what we feel is distinctive and valuable about a psychoanalytic approach as it has developed over time in the public sector. We then ask whether the coming reorganisation is just the latest in an ongoing series of challenges in the NHS, or whether there are grounds for concern about the place of psychoanalytic thinking within the planned service arrangements and within our collective understanding of the nature of psychological development and mental health. This chapter was written towards the end of 2015. While some details may have changed, it seeks to place psychoanalytic psychotherapy with children within a longer time-scale and in relation to fundamental issues.

Psychoanalytic thinking played a significant role in the beginnings of mental health services for children and adolescents in the UK. This was initially through its general influence on clinical thinking at that time, and, subsequently, through the presence within these services of psychoanalytically trained clinicians and their application of a psycho-analytic approach to the needs of different patient groups in changing circumstances. In the post-war social and intellectual climate in which the NHS came into being, and in which thinking about childhood was informed by innovators like John Bowlby and Donald Winnicott, an NHS training in child psychotherapy, based on the observation of chil-dren in ordinary as well as clinical settings, was established. At the same time, an observational approach to the study of infancy and to clinical teaching and learning more broadly was developed at what was then the Tavistock Centre through the work of Esther Bick, Martha Harris, and Isca Salzberger-Wittenberg and colleagues (Harris Williams, 2011; Salzberger-Wittenberg et al., 1983). Since then, three voluntary sector trainings and a second NHS training school have been established across England and Scotland. In recent years, a number of trainings to work psychotherapeutically with children have emerged, but the focus of this chapter is limited to the work of those who trained through the NHS-funded schemes accredited by the Association of Child Psychotherapists.

The training and practice of child psychotherapists seeks to balance the claims of two perspectives: an epistemic perspective, that of psychoanalysis, and a practical, ethical perspective, that of a public sector service. As other contributors to this volume make clear, there can be a fruitful relationship between these two perspectives but there are also inherent tensions between them. The commitment to being in the public sector has meant that child psychotherapy has always been subject to changing public concerns and economic reali-ties; the profession is itself part of that public culture. This chapter examines the current situation and its implications for the place of psychoanalytic/psychodynamic thinking within mental health services for children, young people, and their families. (Although the terms are sometimes used interchangeably, we have chosen to use the more specific term psychoanalytic in the rest of the chapter, with its link to the practice of psychoanalysis, rather than the more generic designation psychodynamic, which might be understood as indicating a general understanding of a quality of the mind.)

The development of mental health services for children and adolescents

The multi-disciplinary services within which child psychotherapy became established have undergone many transformations, some of them reflected in the changes of name from Child Guidance to Child and Family Services, and, latterly, Child and Adolescent Mental Health Services (CAMHS). These names trace the move from a more general concern with children's lives and the different ways in which difficulties might be manifested towards a specific concern with mental health and, more recently, to a narrower focus on diagnosable mental disorders. The professional disciplines that made up the teams changed as psychiatric social workers were withdrawn to the local authority and the link with educational psychology largely disappeared. More recently, the teams have expanded from psychiatry, clinical psychology, family and systemic psychotherapy, and child psychotherapy to include nurses, other therapists, and generic mental health workers. Within these teams, forms of consultation and brief intervention emerged out of the different theoretical frameworks of psychoanalytic, systemic, and cognitive thinking.

The core specialist contribution of child psychotherapists to the services they worked in remained that of making individual psycho-analytic psychotherapy a part of the public sector response to those children and adolescents whose current functioning and future lives have been most seriously compromised, whether through vulnerability arising from early relational stress and/or loss, through innate developmental difficulties, or as a result of traumatic and abusive experiences. The psychoanalytic observational study of early mother–infant relationships (Bick, 1964; Miller et al., 1989) as the foundation of the mind's capacity for experience and reflection opened up an avenue to understanding and treating children in local authority care (Boston, 1980; Emanuel, 2002) and those on the autistic spectrum and their parents and carers (Alvarez & Reid, 1999; Rhode & Klauber, 2004) where there had been serious failure in early relationships or a primary developmental difficulty, respectively. It also created a framework for developing a brief therapeutic response to the more ordinary distress and threatened derailments of development in the relationship of under-fives to their parents (Miller, 1992) or of adolescents to their own emerging independent identity (Copley & Forryan, 1997; Waddell, 2002[1998]).

At the time, these clinical developments were not characterised in a way that emphasised their difference from what went before, as perhaps they would be now. Rather, they continued to be termed "psychoanalytic" in that they drew on a model of the mind and of mental functioning which stresses the importance of emotional relationships, both externally and inwardly elaborated as states of mind, and the unconscious nature of much of our mental lives. These clinical developments were also "psychoanalytic" in the sense that they were applications and adaptations of a form of clinical observation and thinking about emotional states as accessible through the therapeutic relationship. This was the foundation of the view that the capacity to do brief clinical work was acquired during training through supervised experience of more extended clinical encounters in which there was time for the complexity of a relationship to unfold. There were no separate, free-standing trainings in these new clinical developments; rather, these different applications of a core way of working were incorporated within the professional training in psychoanalytic psychotherapy with children and adolescents, disseminated to qualified child psychotherapists through workshops, supervision, and study days, and shared with colleagues from a range of work settings through informal consultation and supervision. The assumptions that lay behind such an un-market-oriented view of service development seem anachronistic now but were once widely shared. With the arrival of evidence based practice (EBP) in mental health (Roth & Fonagy, 1996) this situation changed: a new generation of evidence-based "brand name" treatments and related trainings came into being. Just as behavioural therapies were designed for experimental research, so these new interventions met the new demands of EBP, because they were designed to do so. It has been much harder for those treatments, such as psychoanalytic psychotherapy, that emerged out of clinical practice prior to this change to develop a research methodology appropriate to the nature of the treatment offered and to gain the funding needed for an evidence base. There was inevitably a delay before a randomised control trial (RCT) could be established for psychoanalytic psychotherapy, both for treatment resistant depression in adults (Tavistock Adult Depression Study: Fonagy et al., 2015; Taylor et al., 2012) and for the treatment of moderate to severe depression in adolescents. Short-term psychoanalytic psychotherapy (STPP) is one arm of an RCT, the IMPACT study, which is due to start reporting back in 2016

(Midgley et al., 2013). (An earlier research study (Trowell et al., 2007) on childhood depression was critiqued because it lacked, for ethical reasons, a control group.)

During the period between the 1970s and early 2000s, child psychotherapists (now increasingly called child and adolescent psychotherapists) built a place for psychoanalytic clinical work within the public sector. The multi-disciplinary team was seen as the appropriate setting for treating children and young people (even where the treatment is undertaken in private practice, it is assumed that this multi-disciplinary perspective and the external context of care will be kept in mind by the clinician). Providing mental health services within the framework of limited public resources was considered to be a shared team task, and as a result of the demands of this setting there was a continuing development of psychoanalytically based interventions that address the needs of those for whom individual psychotherapy, as traditionally understood, is not appropriate or acceptable. In 1999, Alan Shuttleworth wrote of the necessity for child and adolescent psychotherapists to inhabit a "dual nationality" in CAMHS teams, providing work of a standard that is recognised both by the psychoanalytic and by public sector communities, contributing to the more generic functions of CAMHS teams as well as to the specialist treatment of the most severe and entrenched mental health difficulties and disorders. This need to find a balance can also be thought of in terms of the claims of external facts—of the patient's history, current symptoms, and circumstances—and an attention to the way those facts are lived out in the present within the imagination, within patterns of feeling and ways of relating, and within family narratives. Managing this balance enabled child and adolescent psychotherapists to develop a distinctive disciplinary contribution to CAMHS teams. This meant that when national standards for child health and social care were drawn up in 2004, the profession was included as a core profession within multi-disciplinary child and adolescent mental health teams (Department of Health, 2004).

The CAMHS transformation as a service reorganisation

In the ten years since the National Service Framework, the long-term mismatch between the resourcing of mental health services for both adults and children and the ever-increasing demands made on them has become a public crisis. Within CAMHS, there have been efforts to manage this resource gap by cutting staffing costs, both in terms of absolute numbers and by stripping out more senior clinical posts, which may create a recruitment and retention problem for the future, and by raising thresholds for accessing services. In parallel with concern about resources, there has been mounting anxiety about the mental health of children and young people, and about high rates of depression, anxiety, and self-harm in particular, culminating in the CAMHS Review (2014) and the Department of Health's *Future in Mind* (2015), which lays out the vision and mechanisms for CAMHS transformation over the next five years.

The aims of this transformation—of increasing access to collaboratively organised services that offer evidence-based treatments delivered in a way that is transparent and respectful of service users and attentive to their experience—are ones with which no one could possibly disagree. This, however, does raise the question of what it might be about the nature of the task itself that such uncontentious aims have apparently proved so difficult to achieve. The document does not examine this issue but sets out a national reorganisation of CAMHS as the solution. Moreover, there are other unaddressed issues that may become more apparent with the passage of time. In particular, the "evidence base" is inevitably not a zone of pure science separate from the political and financial pressures that determine the allocation of research funding (Kennedy, 2015), while the aims of the CAMHS transformation have emerged in a context of cumulative changes that have been under way within the culture of CAMHS and public services generally for some time.

By this, we mean that there has been a shift away from the involvement of clinicians, in any substantial and meaningful sense, in issues of service planning, which has led to an increasing gap between a business management approach and the complexity and chronicity that are characteristic of most CAMHS referrals. There is a pressure within such an approach to see mental health problems as requiring technical solutions, in the form of specific packages of intervention delivered without the need either to establish a relational context for treatment, or to "take account of the clinical heterogeneity found within diagnostic categories and . . . a more personalised approach to treatment" (Kennedy, 2015). A view of evidence as established exclusively through

RCTs, such that other forms of evidence have been excluded, and the disproportion in UK mental health research funding between CBT (27.55%) and psychodynamic psychotherapy (1.96%) (Kennedy, 2015), has had a profound impact on clinicians, managers, and commissioners and on the kind of mental health treatments that are now available on the ground.

Alongside these changes there has been the introduction of a new approach to clinical work and service organisation, which aims not only to manage service capacity more effectively but to transform mental health services for children and young people in line with the earlier transformation that IAPT (Improving Access to Psychological Therapies) brought to adult mental health services in 2006. (For a critical appraisal, see McQueen, 2009.) In 2011, Children and Young People's IAPT (CYP-IAPT) was established as a service transformation programme delivered by NHS England with the aim of bringing a standardisation of services in terms of therapeutic interventions, outcome monitoring, and workforce development. However, given the disproportion in research funding and the skewed nature of the evidence available, there is a concern that the configuration of CAMHS will become fixed around the existing evidence base: CBT for anxiety and depression, Parent Training for conduct disorder, Systemic Family Practice for conduct disorder, depression, and self-harm, and Interpersonal Psychotherapy for Adolescents with depression (IPT-A). This will make it difficult to maintain a space for psychoanalytically informed modalities of treatment, whatever might be the outcome of the IMPACT study (Midgley et al., 2013). There is a risk that, with the shortage of funding for both research and clinical services, the door will close on further developments, particularly those involving longer-term interventions for more severe and enduring conditions, which are inevitably more expensive and ethically complicated to research

The CAMHS transformation as a new paradigm

There is an argument that the crisis in CAMHS that the CAMHS transformation is intended to solve is not solely due to resource pressures. Neither is it due to the unwillingness of professionals to engage with the realities of service delivery, the need for transparency as to outcomes and research (Midgley et al., 2009), and for national clinical standards. Rather, it is the consequence of a broader failure to understand the nature of the mental health task. Timimi (2015) writes of the impact on the ground of a "medico-technical" model of interventions, which leaves no space for perspectives on mental health that are concerned with "relationships, contexts and values". Whatever the intention of policy-makers, the way in which effort and funding is targeted means that a clinical approach that seeks to integrate developmental, affective, relational, and contextual elements is being replaced by a "technical", symptom-based, problem-solving approach that bypasses the need to assess the particular context of a patient's difficulties and a consideration of the therapeutic relationship (Timimi, 2015). It seems that children's mental health services are following those for adults, where considerations of service-user preference, clinical judgement, and individualised treatment have been replaced by a stepped care model and a bias towards guided self-care and CBT in the guidelines on adult depression, despite the evidence to the contrary contained within the guidelines themselves (McQueen, 2009; McQueen & St John Smith, 2015). The term service user rather than patient is linked to a larger debate about perceptions of mental health services, but is sometimes taken to imply a responsiveness and transparency to user views that is not borne out in these recent developments. Partly for this reason, we have avoided this term and, where possible, refer to parents, children, and adolescents.

It is unclear whether there is evidence that such symptom-focused interventions can produce sustainable improvement in patients presenting with serious, long-standing, multi-dimensional conditions which are "influenced by a myriad of [sic] contextual factors" (Kennedy, 2015). Neither is it clear that a symptom-focused approach can support a sufficiently complex account of the needs of most CAMHS patients or the needs of CAMHS teams, so that a workforce can be developed and retained whose training and experience is adequate to the assessment and treatment of that level of disturbance. The need to classify by manifest symptoms on referral is necessary for basic data collection and auditing but, for an understanding of the patient's predicament and for research into the nature of the therapeutic relationship, one also needs a model that can accommodate complex processes, which take place outside of awareness and conscious control. The lack of this dimension has led to a conception of the therapeutic process as being overly conscious and cognitive and, therefore, emotionally and relationally unproblematic. Shedler (2010) describes, in relation to adult mental health in the USA, the way in which an uncritical acceptance of the early research into CBT led to an over-inflation of the claims for this particular model of the mind, at the expense of an appreciation of the relational dimension that under-lies all successful interventions including CBT (though this is not recognised within the treatment model itself). The argument he makes with respect to CBT—that the more the clinician adheres to the manual, rather than being able to draw on their experience of a ther-apeutic relationship, the less successful the outcome—might well hold true for other treatments. If so, it follows that what is needed within CAMHS is the capacity to create and sustain a therapeutic relation-ship under difficult circumstances, a capacity acquired slowly with the support of more experienced clinicians. However, those currently involved in CYP-IAPT training are given an impression that is quite the opposite of Shedler's argument: that what is required is adherence to the manual, and that such manualised interventions can be taught to, and delivered by, a less well trained and, therefore, cheaper work-force. While some services will still have experienced clinicians who can support and supervise these less well trained colleagues, career structures have been stripped out, and it must follow that, over time, CAMHS will increasingly become staffed by people trained to imple-ment a manual rather than to struggle with the challenges of estab-lishing a therapeutic relationship in a way that engages and develops them over a professional career.

Clinical thinking and the therapeutic relationship

Those referred to CAMHS have complex difficulties. Precisely because the number of clinical appointments offered is limited, an approach is needed that enables the clinician to focus on the way the individual or family expresses their difficulties. That attention to the complexity implicit in whatever the person is communicating needs to be available as much in a single meeting as over a number of sessions; it needs to inform clinical judgement alongside the "facts" of the history and external context. For this, the clinician needs a capac-ity to observe not only what is being said, but also what is not being said and the feelings that accompany it, whether they are expressed by the person seeking help or experienced only by the clinician.

The complexity of an individual child, adolescent, or parent's predicament could well be concealed in borrowed, pre-processed phrases that package the problem in misleadingly general terms—for example, "He's attention-seeking". The clinical task is to find a way to enable a more personal expression of the situation, in this case a particular mother and child's feelings about each other. Being helped to re-engage with what is happening and to find a way of expressing afresh, and more fully, what had been just a thing-like formulation ("He's attention-seeking") is itself therapeutic. However, the predicament that needs to be understood might not be available for expression verbally at all, but only through a style of behaving, the atmosphere this creates in the room, and the feelings evoked in the clinician.

Thus, a very troubled and troubling young person referred to CAMHS seemed unable to tell the psychotherapist who saw her for an initial meeting what was on her mind. However, she had communicated something important about her state through arriving too early and having to wait, while also managing to hide herself away so that the clinic receptionist was unaware of her presence until the time of the appointment had passed. Such a young person could easily find herself dropped by a hard-pressed service because, before anything else could be offered to her, she needed someone to notice her angry preoccupation with being disregarded, something that at first she could only enact rather than speak about. Even more likely to get lost is the mute depression of an adolescent who habitually manages any painful feelings by cutting off their mental awareness and cutting into their skin. To make contact with such a young person, one cannot rely on their capacity to express need, but only on what is noticed and felt by the clinician in their presence. Within this model of clinical work, it is only by experiencing the clinician as paying thoughtful attention to whatever is presented as being a communication, and, thereby, transforming it into communication, that the individual is helped to take himself seriously, to become more self-observant, and eventually to find within his own mind a sustainable way of living his life. Such an approach is especially needed by those whose difficulties are less specific, more pervasive, and more longstanding and who are not likely to be helped by forms of intervention that require a greater degree of awareness of the nature of the problem and a capacity to engage straightforwardly with whatever help is offered. A critical review of the research found psychodynamic psychotherapy with children and adolescents to be effective across a range of different conditions, indicating that the establishment of a relationship with the young person might be more salient than the diagnosis (Midgley & Kennedy, 2011).

The complexities of an individual's difficulties are always present within a clinical encounter, whether one attends to them or not. If, through a need to follow a treatment protocol, that complexity is overlooked, the result is both a loss of understanding about the individual's predicament and, much more serious, the creation for that person of an experience of not being heard. Attending to the particular qualities of an encounter does not necessarily imply a protracted treatment, but it is crucial to any successful intervention precisely because the absence of such an experience—of being the object of someone else's care and attention—characterises the psychological development of many, if not most, of those referred to CAMHS. The severity of depression and anxiety among those referred bespeaks early-established patterns of difficulty, whether due to subtle failures in the fabric of reciprocity and relatedness at the start of life, innate developmental deficits, or a serious dysfunction of the parenting environment. In place of the unfolding of ordinary development, one sees instead the emergence of unhelpful, self-defeating, and self-destructive ways of coping with states of feeling that have gone un-minded and unrecognised. Central to this conception of an intervention is the relationship between the person struggling to express her predicament, in whatever way she can, and the person whose task is to notice and think about the kind of relationship that is forming in the room—a task that must take place before there is any possibility of the person referred for help being able to take responsibility for her own need and wish to change.

The approach we are describing is not the sole preserve of psychoanalytic clinicians, but the difficulties in, and impediments to, sustaining a therapeutic relationship, and the way this relationship refracts the emotional qualities of formative relationships that have been internalised early in development, have been central elements in psychoanalytic thinking. While the hope for change may be sustained by helpful aspects of a child or young person's experience, the legacy of fragile or failed relationships that have undermined and distorted their capacities will need to find a home. The therapeutic relationship cannot, therefore, be a straightforwardly "good" one. It needs to include, and to be able to cope with, the anxiety and anger of difficult and destructive experiences, and the clinician will need to assume responsibility for the maintenance of the contact in the face of difficulties and disruptions, rather than relying on an expressed wish for help. For this, the clinician needs to have a reliable setting, temporarily safe from the anxieties and pressures on the team outside, and sufficient training to be able to remain thoughtful and realistic while, at the same time, sustaining receptiveness to the states of unreachability, anger, or despair that are being communicated. While the aim of such an approach is to allow something more hopeful and resilient to emerge, its value might also lie in creating an understanding of the individual's functioning as the basis for planning of future interventions, perhaps of a quite different kind.

There is a clear difference between a "technical" model of treatment and one based on a therapeutic relationship as a focus for observing external and internalised relationships. An intervention that depends on the establishing of a relationship, and on the gradual coming into awareness of failed patterns of relating, is inherently open-ended and uncertain. Paradoxically, however, this reliance on the therapeutic relationship is linked to the long-term generative potential of that intervention after treatment has ended: the "sleeper effect", which has been reported in research into psychoanalytic modalities of treatment and which can be understood within the terms of the model itself (Trowell et al., 2007). In ordinary development, the mind grows through internalising and identifying with the qualities of the first relationships; in treatment, what is offered is an experience of a relationship that can contain states of feeling that could not be managed in the past. Identification with the qualities of the therapeutic relationship creates the internal emotional basis for continuing development.

Child and adolescent psychotherapists in CAMHS

The contribution that psychoanalytic thinking can make to a CAMHS, both directly through clinical work and indirectly through participation in a team, is dependent on the overall culture in a service. It is harder to demonstrate the value of such an approach in those CAMHS where senior clinicians of all disciplines have been replaced by less experienced staff, who have been tasked with implementing discrete, pre-existing packages of manualised interventions, without the need to keep in mind and take account of the multi-dimensional nature of most referrals.

At the time of writing, the CAMHS service in Leicester had undergone various reconfigurations in response to the rise in referral numbers, but it had so far resisted the pressure towards an IAPT model of discrete, symptom-based assessments and interventions. Following a recent service evaluation, various models of practice for CAMHS were considered, including CAPA (Choice and Partnership Appointments). While Leicester CAMHS adopted those elements of this approach that supported realistic service planning, it retained a multi-disciplinary input to most initial assessments through a team discussion between other clinicians with different approaches and levels of experience, including child psychotherapists. It has also maintained a balance between generic and specialist interventions in the clinical workload of all disciplines. This is particularly important for child psychotherapists, who need to be seen to be contributing to managing the rising referral rates; it also avoids a split between clinicians whose task is to meet the needs of those who can be helped by a brief initial intervention and those members of the team who are engaged in longer-term work with complex and intractable problems.

The clinical contribution of child and adolescent psychotherapists

Some children and young people with serious mental health problems need substantial interventions, including psychoanalytic psychotherapy, and some might be referred for psychotherapy directly after an initial assessment. However, it is equally important that other members of the team feel able to refer children and adolescents where concerns remain after other interventions have been tried and failed. A recent audit in Leicester CAMHS found that those referred to child psychotherapy had had, on average, 2.54 previous unsuccessful interventions. This appears to be in line with other services (Keenan et al., 2013), and indicates the importance of having psychoanalytic psychotherapy as a treatment available within a CAMHS team, even though it is often not the first intervention to be offered. However, this requires both an atmosphere within a team and a management stance that can accommodate and recognise when an intervention is insufficient and support a longer-term treatment without, of course, the certainty of a better outcome. The IMPACT study (Midgely et al., 2013) has reported on the efficacy of short-term psychoanalytic psychotherapy (STPP). The example below shows how this form of treatment was able to reach a young person, aspects of whose mental life had become very split off. The care and collaboration of different members of the team provided the context in which psychotherapy could take place.

A sixteen-year-old girl, Emma, who had been known to CAMHS since she was fourteen, presented with depression and some features of anxiety. Initially, she was offered psychiatric review appointments and referred for CBT. She appeared to engage with this twelve-session intervention and was discharged from the service after about four months. Six months later, Emma was re-referred with an increase in depressive symptoms. On this occasion she was also prescribed anti-depressant medication and offered a more extended period of CBT; when, after twenty sessions, her depression had not lifted, she was offered twenty-eight weekly sessions of STPP over nine months. In the course of treatment it was possible to see, in the relationship she formed with the psychotherapist, something of the complex processes that underlay Emma's depression and anxiety. The traumatic loss of her father in early childhood had not been lived through at the time in a way that allowed the anger, helplessness, and sadness resulting from this loss to be gradually faced and assimilated as one might have expected, in part because of her mother's fragility and depression. Emma coped instead by becoming compliant on the surface, disowning her own emotional state to an extent that eventually became unsustainable. Helping Emma meant observing, as something happening in real time in the room, the way she split off feelings she could not deal with, and finding ways to talk to her about the anxiety she felt about the fragility and unreliability of others, including her psychotherapist, which made this splitting necessary. The inevitable separations and losses that occurred within the therapeutic relationship became opportunities for her to re-experience in a more manageable way what had once been an intolerable sense of abandonment and loss (of father and, indirectly, of mother). Over time, she recovered an awareness of her feelings of anger and helplessness. This enabled her to regain a sense of agency and to re-engage with an adolescent world, returning to college. By the end of this treatment, she no longer required medication.

The levels of disturbance which are associated with neglectful, cruel, and perverse early care both undermine and distort development in ways that do not lend themselves to ordinary diagnostic categories and the symptom-focused interventions of many CAMHS. There is a long history of child psychotherapists working with children in the care system who have endured these sorts of experiences, though access to psychotherapy is affected by local arrangements between CAMHS and Children's Social Care. Young people in kinship care have often survived similar neglect and abuse. Being placed in the care of family members can be a hopeful development, but this does not take away the impact of early trauma, and the painfulness of the family dynamics can compromise the placement. Yet, this additional complexity is often overlooked by services and, since they are not formally considered as "looked-after" children, less support is available both for them and their new carers.

Such children and young people might be referred to CAMHS with presentations of hyperactivity, anxiety, behaviour problems, and difficulties that may be seen as indicative of depression, but the immediate symptoms need to be understood in the light of the experiences they have lived through. In ongoing clinical work, it becomes clear that, when working with a young person with such a history, you are trying to form a relationship with someone who is living in "multiple families in their mind" (Rustin, 1999), oscillating between different internal representations of relationships, which mirror multiple external experiences, past and present. Thus, a young person, who might appear at first to relate in an ordinary, straightforward way, requesting help and hoping that help can be offered, might suddenly lose any faith in the interaction or might even respond to the therapist as someone who is causing harm or making a sadistic attack. There has to be time for a slow, careful, and repeated examination of the communication if some understanding of these triggers is to be achieved. The challenge that these families bring to a CAMHS is not limited to the psychotherapy room, but often extends to the service as a whole. Other members of staff, the receptionist, and the fabric and facilities of the building, which can be experienced at times as an idealised place, can also, following a shut door, a toy missing from the toy box, or a missed appointment, become the site for an acute re-experience of parental failure. Parallel (and, in many cases, joint) work with the carers of the referred child is essential to create a stable and meaningful context for the treatment, addressing painful issues in the shared family history so that a space can be made for the young person to grow into an individual in his or her own right. However, such work involves a CAMHS team committing considerable clinical effort over time and coping with the anxieties associated with failure, or a limited degree of success, because not to do so means allowing the damage inflicted in the past to be carried over into the future. This takes a clinical service outside the apparent certainties of diagnostic pathways and the apparent assurance of following the evidence-based manualised treatments for that diagnosis.

The experience of psychoanalytic psychotherapy with children and adolescents has generated an approach to working with parents and families that is significantly different from what is offered by conventional forms of parenting training (Rustin, 1999). Rather, it is a clinical intervention that seeks to understand a parent's state of mind and its implications for how they receive and manage, or fail to manage, the feelings their children stir up in them and the likely link to their own experience of being parented.

The mother of a paediatric patient was having difficulty supporting her son with his painful, life-long condition. She seemed manic and out of touch with both her child's needs and her own state. However, her response to an initial appointment and the clinician questioning whether everything was, as she claimed, fine, was a sudden collapse. She readily accepted further meetings, in the course of which she became increasingly aware of, and slowly reflective about, her state of confusion and depression. Her own childhood had been chaotic and neglectful and earlier attempts by her GP to help her by prescribing medication or referring her to IAPT appointments had failed. When her first IAPT therapist left after three appointments, this mother found herself unable to manage the steps required to start again with someone else. Similarly, she found it impossible to sustain an awareness of needing to see her GP about medication long enough to actually arrange an appointment. It became apparent that the loss of the IAPT therapist, and the need to negotiate with a receptionist in order to see her GP, only reawakened her abandonment as a young child into the inadequate care of a relative, and her subsequent mode of surviving by putting on what she called her "mask". Although the meetings with the child psychotherapist were not sufficient in themselves, they brought this mother to a more realistic appreciation of her difficulties and her need for a referral for appropriate help, as well as enabling her to see and respond to her child's difficulties less as a meaningless persecution and more as an indication that he was alive to his own need for her parenting. By taking the extent of this mother's predicament seriously, contact with her became possible. Even if she had not been able to respond to this experience, this approach allowed the clinician to understand the nature and extent of the problem that underlay her child's refusal of treatment. As such, it offers a way of working with birth parents who are struggling with a difficult child, foster and adoptive parents trying to manage a traumatised child, or a kinship carer, who has, in addition, to manage the practical and emotional situation of being a member of the same family as the neglectful or abusive birth parent. Whether as a piece of clinical work in its own right or in support of a child in psychotherapy, such work addresses the transgenerational issues that contribute to the intractable nature of the difficulties with which children present in CAMHS. It is work on the interface between adult and children's services, but it can be effective with a level of difficulty that is serious in terms of its impact on the next generation but for which resources are generally not available in adult mental health teams.

Contributing to building and sustaining a CAMHS team

The kind of attention to the particularity and complexity of mental health difficulties that is offered in a sustained way to individual children and young people in psychotherapy is helpful in the range of encounters with those referred to CAMHS. It is also supportive of clinical teams in their challenging and often stressful encounters with those referred for help. While maintaining a direct clinical service to children, young people, and their families, child and adolescent psychotherapists in Leicestershire CAMHS have been able to develop a broader role in supporting the work of their professional colleagues. This role would once have been generally assumed to be a responsibility of more senior clinicians within CAMHS towards less experienced colleagues and Tier 1 professionals, but recent changes have made this work quite unusual. Its purpose is not to compete with other theoretical frameworks but, rather, to help develop the capacity within the team to keep the emotional encounter, and the ability to reflect on it, at the heart of their work. This is especially important in the current climate. While there is turbulence inherent in the emotional states stirred up in clinical work that can "disrupt and distort professional practice" (Rustin, 2008), there is also a pressure to simplify and routinise the clinical encounter, which generates optimistic but unsustainable goals at odds with facing the difficult realities of the task. An unintended but unfortunate outcome of such optimistic goal setting can be to devalue the merits of a steady engagement with the difficulties inherent in clinical work, through which, over time, experience can be developed, retained, and built on within teams.

Alongside offering staff individual supervision and consultation, this kind of steady thinking has been promoted in Leicester CAMHS through the introduction of "work discussion groups". These are facilitated by child psychotherapists, whose task is to help keep the focus on the details of the clinical encounter with patients and the feelings evoked by it, so that the group can be helped to think about what the patient is trying to communicate. This follows the model for developing an observation-based capacity for clinical thinking in the training of child psychotherapists. Work discussion groups are a particular kind of reflective practice group, whereby regular discussions of clinical work take place among small, stable groups of professional workers. Such groups have been highlighted as models of good practice (Department for Education and Skills/Department of Health, 2006).

Working at the margins: psychoanalytic work with adolescents in the voluntary sector

Open Door is a voluntary sector service for young people. Since it was set up forty years ago, the service has drawn on psychoanalytic thinking for an understanding of the specific nature of adolescent development, for the design of its therapeutic services, and to help contain the high levels of anxiety generated by its young service users, not only in parents and carers, but also in the clinical and non-clinical staff striving to help them. Open Door provides an example of the relevance of psychoanalytic thinking to the complex, clinical needs of this high-risk, often ambivalent, and hard to engage patient population. Despite limited and fluctuating financial resources and the particular funding challenges of the voluntary sector, careful data collection, user involvement, and innovative projects have meant that Open Door has managed to convince not only charitable trusts and individual donors but also commissioners from the NHS and local authority that this approach works and is worth investing in. Yet, this hitherto successful psychoanalytic model of working is now coming up against the very different assumptions of the IAPT model being rolled out in CAMH services nationwide, including those working in the voluntary sector.

Open Door is situated in Haringey, home to some of the most affluent, but also some of the most deprived, communities in London. Its main base is situated in discreet shop-front premises in Crouch End. In the aftermath of the Tottenham riots in 2011, Open Door secured funds as part of the local regeneration initiative and, in 2013, established a new service in the heart of Tottenham, based in a community "enterprise hub" housing start-up businesses and youth training schemes. Each year, Open Door works with around 250 young people (age 12–24) and 120 parents who are concerned about their teenage and young adult children, many of whom are reluctant to engage with services themselves. Nearly seventy per cent of young people self-refer, while professionals can refer under-18s via the single point of access for Haringey CAMHS. Open Door straddles Tiers 2 and 3, though the majority of cases fall within Tier 3 in terms of complexity and risk—more than forty per cent of service-users report self-harm and suicidal ideation and nearly seventy per cent present with depression and anxiety in the moderate to severe clinical range.

Open Door works in partnership with CAMHS, Adult Mental Health Services, and Social Care, as appropriate, to manage risk and ensure safeguarding. It offers psychoanalytic psychotherapy on a brief, medium, and longer-term basis, ranging from a few sessions of crisis work to two years of once-weekly psychotherapy and a small number of three-times-weekly psychotherapy offered by child psychotherapy trainees. Open Door provides clinical placements for NHS funded trainees undertaking child psychotherapy trainings at the Tavistock Clinic and the British Psychotherapy Foundation. CBT and mindfulness-based therapy are also available, often alongside psychotherapy. Adolescents, particularly in the younger age range, can be seen jointly with parents as part of their treatment. Bespoke therapy services are also commissioned by mainstream and special secondary schools. While Open Door is offering an increasing range of therapeutic interventions delivered by a diverse range of clinicians, child psychotherapy remains the core profession within the service, as it has been over the past two decades. A thorough knowledge of child development and a capacity to build therapeutic relationships with young people at different developmental stages across the age range, while remaining attentive to the unconscious phenomena being played out in this relationship, are just some of the distinctive competences equipping child psychotherapists to work effectively with this challenging patient group.

Open Door uses audit, evaluation, and service-user feedback as well as the psychoanalytic thinking of the clinical team to review and develop clinical interventions. One such development is Open Door's brief therapy model for adolescents and young adults. It involves a three-session assessment followed by between twelve and twenty sessions of psychotherapy. Here, the time limit is not simply a response to resource pressures, it is built on clinical experience. It allows the emergence of a preoccupation with endings, separations, and the passing of time that has particular pertinence for adolescents at the transition from childhood to adulthood. However, it is not the time limitedness *per se* that helps these concerns to become available for reflection; it is the particular way of using the clinical relationship to observe the emotional states the young person is struggling with, and enabling these states to emerge as feelings and thoughts that can be recognised and owned, that is central to a psychoanalytic approach.

While Open Door is commissioned by Haringey NHS CCG to provide a Tier 3 service for 12–18-year-olds, which accounts for approximately a third of its financial turnover, significant funding is received from charitable trusts (Comic Relief, BBC Children in Need, Lottery, etc.) and is awarded on a project by project basis by funders insisting on "new ideas". Open Door has been successful in using this to develop projects that address the needs of the particular population it serves while coherently rooting them in a psychoanalytic view of personality development. From this perspective, each stage of development from dependent infant to mature adult brings with it not only gains but losses. It is the successful negotiation of each of these, and the role of parental adults in this, that lays the foundation for future healthy enough development. However, many of the young people who seek help might have their own inherent vulnerabilities as well as having had difficult early experiences that did not provide an adequate basis for this process of development. Thus, a request for help can rarely be met by the straightforward framing of goals; it is, rather, an opportunity to bring into a relationship with an adult some preoccupations that are not easily grasped and recognised. Feelings of judgement, humiliation, and a conscious or unconscious fear of the emergence of more dependent feelings can prove unbearable; hoping for something better mobilises a painful awareness of past failures. By careful attention to the emotional atmosphere, the therapist tries to enable the young person to feel understood and avoid a sudden withdrawal from therapy, resulting in the loss of an opportunity to help the young person find a way of living with ambivalence and separation, dependence and independence.

Open Door has developed a range of responses to the young person and their parents. The effectiveness of the different therapeutic models is based on a psychoanalytic understanding of adolescent development and key aspects of child psychotherapy technique— attentiveness to both conscious and unconscious phenomena through the close and detailed observation of the transference relationship. Perhaps this is best illustrated by a brief description of the assessment phase of a young person who took part in the brief therapy pilot.

Kyra was seventeen when she referred herself to Open Door. She reported "vomiting for no reason": it was not self-induced, and the fear of it preoccupied her to such an extent that she was finding it difficult to do anything. At her first assessment appointment, Kyra smiled nervously at her therapist when she was collected from the waiting room. She was rather underweight, wore no make-up, and was dressed androgynously, keeping her jacket buttoned up throughout. Kyra lived with her parents and younger brother. She was finding it increasingly difficult to attend school and it was hard for her to eat for fear of vomiting, but she felt unable to talk to her parents about the extent of her difficulties, saying that her mother "wouldn't understand—we don't do feelings".

Kyra's distressed accounts of her ruminations about vomiting and her difficulties in leaving her bedroom were accompanied by stiff-lipped declarations that she was "a happy person" who did not know why she was here, who did not want therapy as it would "make it worse". Although she had sought help, it was important to enable her to feel that her ambivalence was acceptable. She eventually agreed to return for another appointment.

In the second session, Kyra's taut smile soon gave way to tears, which this time she could not control. She spoke about her increasing difficulties motivating herself in the morning; she had lost interest in everything. She spoke of a "deep sadness", which she could not explain. She said she had felt a little better after the first session but began to "dread" coming back—she did not want to think about anything but wanted to "cut off" her head and "stop thinking". Still in a state of tearful distress, she said that after the first session she remembered when the vomiting had started—after she saw her friend kissing a boy they both liked and whom they agreed neither would pursue. While she said she was "over it" and the relationship between the boy and her friend did not develop, she had been left with feelings of acute anxiety and nausea. She went on to talk about her hatred of her body, how, unlike other girls, she wanted to put on weight, and how she would pull at her small breasts and hips. She agreed that she wanted to feel more "womanly", to develop. As the end of the session approached she became more tearful, saying she did not want therapy, it was making things worse. She bade a tearful farewell and headed towards the toilet saying she had to pull herself together.

There was a shared sense of relief when Kyra returned to the final assessment session in a less distressed state. She spoke about being very affected by the previous meeting but having had a better week. For the first time, the therapist heard about a long-held part-time job and a plan to start driving lessons. While Kyra still felt anxious around food, she had managed to eat more. She told her therapist that, while the difficult feelings were still there, they felt more manageable and she opted to continue in therapy for the twenty weeks within the pilot study.

This vignette illustrates how frightening the maelstrom of adolescence can be for some young people. These were feelings that the therapist had to accept during the assessment without knowing whether Kyra would break off attending. Being able to think about the anxieties about separation, growing up, and sexuality that Kyra was expressing helped the therapist keep her bearings. Kyra seemed to function in an infantile projective way, ridding herself of unwanted feelings by vomiting. She did not want to think about any of it but instead to "cut off" her head and to evacuate her difficult feelings into her therapist. Her comments about her "unavailable" mother, whether realistic or not, conveyed a lack of primary containment, a sense of being left with unbearable feelings. What is also palpable in these initial meetings is fear of regression to a dependent relationship. However, her desperate cry for help, expressed through her uncontrollable tears, met with an experience of being contained by the structure of the assessment, out of which emerged some capacity both to grow up and to accept further help in doing so.

The evaluation of the brief therapy pilot, which is now the main therapeutic intervention at Open Door, was extremely positive. With both completion and clinical improvement rates well above seventy per cent, the model has become one of Open Door's core therapies (Britton, 2008). Similar psychoanalytic models have developed elsewhere and it is hoped that the imminent publication of the IMPACT study will provide an evidence base for short-term psychoanalytic psychotherapy. However, such an intervention requires the framework of a team and a way of working in which initial consultations can lead to assessments for a variety of treatments, some on a longer-term or more intensive basis. As CYP-IAPT gains traction among NHS commissioners, it will be challenging to preserve what is valuable in the experience and thinking that has informed the work of an organisation like Open Door. The constant pressure in the voluntary sector to demonstrate positive outcomes in order to secure funding has meant that Open Door is well versed in routine evaluation and is, in theory at least, well placed to compete in the new world of evidence-based commissioning. However, as this chapter has suggested, the drive towards the standardisation of clinical interventions and outcome indicators in CAMHS might well render other evidence bases and other ways of conceptualising treatment irrelevant.

At the time of writing, Open Door, like other CAMHS providers across the country, is participating in local "CAMHS transformation" and becoming a CYP-IAPT service. This involves additional training for child psychotherapists in IPT-A (interpersonal psychotherapy for adolescents) or CBT, and CYP-IAPT leadership training for managers in order to ensure that the service complies with the model. Given the uncontentious nature of the stated principles of CYP-IAPT, is there any cause for concern?

There is uncertainty whether there will continue to be a space for psychoanalytic thinking as a way of understanding adolescent development and its difficulties, alongside other approaches, and also whether the range of psychoanalytically based interventions (brief, time-limited, and longer-term) that Open Door has successfully offered in the past can be maintained within this new structure. However, Open Door has opted to participate in this transformation in part to protect its NHS funding, and also to ensure that it remains part of discussions around service design and delivery, in the hope that models of work based on psychoanalytic thinking and evidenced by positive outcomes and ongoing research will endure within mainstream public sector thinking.

Conclusion

So, what is the future place of psychoanalytic thinking likely to be within mental health services for children, young people, and their parents? It is hard to know at this point. That there is a crisis in the provision of children's mental health services is clear. However, we have argued that this is not only a crisis of resourcing or organisation, but also a crisis in how mental health and mental health problems are conceived. While the debate continues to be set in terms of symptom-focused interventions and standardised treatment protocols, it will continue to be difficult to argue that what is needed is attention to the context of disturbance, both within the developing personality of the child and within their external relationships. Timimi (2015) aptly designates such a focus as being on "relationships, context and values". Those referred to CAMHS have difficulties that are serious, complex, and of long standing. Interventions based on an understanding of how patterns of disturbance emerge gradually out of a child's inherent vulnerability and self-damaging efforts to adapt to inadequate and abusive early relationships have, however, been increasingly replaced in CAMHS. Treatments now require a capacity in families and young people to respond straightforwardly in their own interests to therapeutic interventions, strategies of self-care, and advice.

There has been a long-term under-funding of research in the area of child mental health, and within that there has been an overwhelming bias in favour of CBT. Moreover, research and the uses to which it is put within CAMHS are not "immune from vested interests more commonly associated with pharmacological treatments" (Kennedy, 2015). This point is a salutary counterbalance to a view of the evidence base as standing outside such vested interests. It calls into question the uncritical acceptance that it should, without further consideration, dictate clinical services. A more cautious use of the evidence would allow a distinction between the levels of need that different interventions are designed to ameliorate and the different scope of didactic, symptom-focused, and relational interventions.

In ordinary development, the human ability to mentalize and reflect on experience—essential to well-being, to the capacity to relate to others, and to parenting—is the internalised outcome of early relationships, of being held in someone else's mind (Bion, 1962; Winnicott, 1960). Parenting is now widely understood to involve subtle capacities for emotional attunement that take place outside of awareness, drawing on the parents' own deeply embrained experiences of having themselves been parented (Fonagy et al., 2003; Hobson, 2002; Trevarthen, 1998). Much could be lost in seeking to transform the fruits of this perspective into techniques that can be taught without the need for an attentive human context, if careful consideration is not also given to which children and families need a relational, rather than didactic, approach to their difficulties.

There is a risk that the skewed nature of the research base and the way its clinical implications are interpreted will create teams that mirror these very limitations, that are better able to engage with the less disturbed and the more motivated. There might well be a gap between the intention of policy-makers and how those policies are implemented locally, but the two levels reinforce each other in a way that makes it difficult for clinicians who disagree to intervene at any level. The CAMHS review (2014) looks to "early intervention" to help stem the rising level of demands on CAMHS. Whatever might have been the intention of policy-makers, this is often understood on the ground as brief interventions suitable to the less troubled, rather than earlier interventions in the life history of very disturbed families.

Unless failures of engagement and patterns of repeated referrals for brief treatment episodes over a childhood are recorded and monitored alongside the immediate outcome measures for completed treatments, we cannot know whether the new configuration of CAMHS is meeting the needs of the most troubled children and families. While it might seem economic to offer repeated short-term interventions, it might not be cost-effective in the long run. It is certainly not without its cost to individual children, young people, and families, who eventually pass out of the system feeling that it is they who have failed, without ever having received help that adequately reflected the seriousness of their needs. It is the needs of this group that child psychotherapists have particularly sought to address.

CHAPTER FOUR

Siobhan O'Connor: two tributes*

Richard Ingram and Carine Minne

Richard Ingram: memories of Siobhan in Northern Ireland

I had the privilege of knowing Siobhan as a friend and colleague for over twenty years, both as a psychiatry trainee and then as a consultant psychiatrist in the NHS in Northern Ireland. She was one of the most vital, effective, and fearless individuals I have encountered in my entire career, and for me, as for many others, she was a powerful and formative influence as well as a generous friend. In her homeland, she made a very major contribution to the development of analytic thinking and practice, which has left both an established legacy and a developing one. This she continued in her work in London at the South London and Maudsley Trust and the Institute of Psychoanalysis, when she left to live there permanently over ten years ago.

Siobhan was first and foremost a doctor—a psychiatrist—and in this way followed in a family tradition, and, of course, it was this foundation as a psychiatrist through which she developed her deep interest

* These tributes were presented at the joint Scientific and Applied Scientific meeting of the Institute of Psychoanalysis on Wednesday 20 May 2015. They were published in the Confidential Institute of Psychoanalysis bulletin. Reprinted with kind permission.

and extensive expertise in psychoanalysis. As the first ever dual trainee in psychotherapy and general psychiatry in Northern Ireland, Siobhan began to develop a key role in providing introductory training in psychoanalysis for psychiatry trainees and other multi-professional staff. Her Wednesday lunchtime lectures in the Albertbridge Road Day Hospital in East Belfast were a sell-out event, with high attendances despite the logistical impediments in place due to the bomb scares and army checkpoints, which at that time regularly brought Belfast traffic to a standstill or turned it into an obstacle course at best. With her powerful presence and strong, broad humour, she cut a fearless figure at local psychiatric conferences, case presentations, and seminars.

A significant attraction of my own first consultant post in Downshire Hospital in Downpatrick was that Siobhan would be my colleague. Having been influenced by her example, like a considerable number of my contemporaries, I had started my own analytic training. I am happy to say this is a tradition that has persisted successfully, and when, a few years ago, Siobhan asked me about the state of interest in analytic training among local trainee psychiatrists, on a quick head count I estimated that around half of all senior trainees in the Belfast training were at least in some level of training analysis—a situation unheard of in any other medical deanery. She did, however, not seem to fully recognise her pivotal and catalytic importance in creating a foundation for this, so I was glad, given subsequent sad developments, to have had an opportunity to put her straight on the contribution she had made.

At the point I joined Siobhan in Downshire, having been given fairly meagre resources, she had already established a small psychotherapy service with a team of group therapists, and spent the rest of her time running a traditional community mental health team. However, when given the opportunity to move full time into psychotherapy, she took things, true to form, in an entirely different but equally productive direction and made a decision to shift her general adult commitment to the most disturbed patients in the hospital—those housed in the locked wards that would be called psychiatric intensive care units (PICUs). This surprised many of her colleagues, as it was probably the most unpopular role in the service; it was also one that few thought a psychoanalyst would have the appropriate skills to manage, as the service had always been heavily biased towards a traditional approach involving drug interventions and behaviourism.

In this setting, her principal aim was the effective application of psychoanalytic principles and treatment in the service of understanding and managing mental health patients who present with very high levels of disturbance, diagnostic complexity, and risk. She realised that, given the lack of resources and analytic awareness in the service, she could offer only a limited volume of direct patient treatment: therefore, she concentrated her efforts on the application of psychoanalytic thinking to the complexities and dynamics within staff teams and the institution of the mental health service responsible for providing care for this patient group.

So, in came a raft of changes, including psychoanalytically orientated supervision for individual staff and group reflective practice. Institutionally orientated supervision was now on offer at staff meetings and other Trust venues, bringing in an awareness of the need to understand the psychopathology of patients and its effects on the service at all levels, from the chief executive to the nursing auxiliary. In terms of individual therapeutic approaches, this was very much orientated towards enabling her patients (the most disturbed in the service) to arrive at a level of awareness of their minds (or indeed help them to discover that they had minds) and their functioning. Through her approach, they were helped to acquire, where possible, an awareness of who they were (including being an individual who is suffering the trauma of realising that he or she has a mental illness), what he or she has done, and what impact this has on the minds of others.

For most staff, her insights brought both relief and disquiet, particularly the understanding of how individual staff and the institution contributed to difficult dynamics that often acted to undermine therapeutic progress. However, it was the measures that she gradually introduced to process and contain the anxieties around such issues, and the positive results that they produced, which carried her programme forward. Such was her influence that, to the present, my colleagues, many of whom spent placements with her as trainees, often and spontaneously recall the impact on them of her interventions and the effects of her capacity to tune into the psychotic frequencies of her patients, through what seemed to be such an effortlessly derived comment or intervention which produced an unexpected but significant therapeutic shift.

Finally, I would like to pay tribute to Siobhan's contribution to the development of the Northern Ireland Association for the Study of

Psychoanalysis (NIASP)—a member institution of the British Psycho-analytic Council—which is a vibrant post-qualification organisation in Northern Ireland for psychoanalysts and psychoanalytic psychother-apists, and a training body for psychoanalytic psychotherapy. NIASP developed from a small group of interested individuals, from a multi-plicity of backgrounds, which coalesced around Thomas Freeman—the only training analyst in Ireland at that time—in the 1980s. The Association came into being formally in 1988 with Siobhan as its inau-gural Chair. It was under her lengthy stewardship, and due to the increasing recognition of its high quality of training, which main-tained a strong emphasis on a four- to five-times weekly training analysis and on establishing training links with psychoanalysts in Great Britain, that NIASP gained its accreditation within the BPC.

NIASP represents the embodiment of a very important part of Siobhan's legacy. Through it, a psychoanalytically knowledgeable community has developed, with NIASP at its centre, unique in the UK and particularly notable in the prevailing context of Northern Ireland. But again, Siobhan's vision and strength of character, as well as her sheer intellectual and professional capability, meant another trail was blazed for the greater good. I—along with many others—have bene-fited personally from this situation and the opportunities it has facili-tated, such as through the former sponsorship training with the Institute of Psychoanalysis in London, by which a group of psycho-analysts has become established in Northern Ireland.

Siobhan's sudden and untimely death is particularly sad as it came at a time in her life when she was full of plans for the future, in partic-ular writing about her experience and work. She remains very much missed by family, friends, and colleagues.

Carine Minne: memories of Siobhan in London

Siobhan was one of those people you felt privileged to know. She was a big character, with a big voice, who had big opinions and was big on compassion. If she had not done medicine and ended up as a psychiatrist–psychoanalyst, I believe she could have been one of those rare politicians with real integrity. She was a mover and shaker. She got things done.

My first memories of meeting Siobhan were in London. I got to know her through a mutual friend, Clare Doherty, another loud psychoanalytic woman from the north of Ireland. These three vocal northern Irish women used to meet up for glasses of wine together, when Siobhan would always hope for a big conflicted discussion about anything really, but the problem was that the three of us used to agree on most things, leaving Siobhan robbed of a good argie-bargie. There were many giggles together and what tended to happen was that, even on topics that we completely agreed on, Siobhan always agreed even louder than Clare or me, somehow managing to make agreement appear problematic! It is truly heartbreaking to think that both Siobhan and Clare have left the planet.

In her world of work, Siobhan used those strong character traits, combined with her psychiatric and psychoanalytic trainings, in the most constructive ways. She loved a challenge. So, for example, in her earlier years, the 1990s, instead of carrying on working as a psychiatrist in the community, she took on the challenge of looking after a locked ward filled with suffering patients and suffering nurses that most other psychiatrists dreaded working on. These disturbed patients, who could not be moved to other wards, or rehabilitated to the community, were frequently violent, and this was managed using high doses of oral and intramuscular neuroleptics along with intermittent short-acting tranquillisers. Her offer to take on this ward was welcomed by her colleagues, who warned her that her wish to change the regime from drug-controlled to a more therapeutic environment would be resisted, by nurses and patients.

What Siobhan observed was that the nurses made demands of her constantly to "do something" and that the patients made demands on the nurses to "do something". The nurses would react with disappointment when she did not produce a magic solution, but the patients reacted with violence when the nurses did not. There were many maladaptive defensive responses to increased times of disturbance on the ward: increasing the drugs given; changing the routines, so that the little art therapy input was cancelled, availability of nurses to be with their nominated patients was cancelled because several nurses were required to control one patient, and the rare escorted leaves off the ward would be cancelled. Everyone ended up even more frustrated—the nurses for realising their neglect of other patients, the art therapist for being made redundant, the patients for seeing that one patient would be getting all the attention, meaning that they would become more disturbed as a response, creating a vicious circle.

Siobhan's task was to break this circle, where pharmacotherapy was idealised but kept failing as a solution. She made use of the concept of mental processes, whereby she described a biological disso-lution of the structures that organise higher mental processes, leaving the more primitive processes to emerge. Where Siobhan excelled was in her ability to consider psychoanalytic concepts as applicable not only to understanding what was going on in the patients, but also in the clinical team itself. Long before true reflective practice "caught on" as essential for the healthy functioning of a psychiatric ward, Siobhan was busy applying her psychoanalytic knowledge on this very diffi-cult ward with a scientific hat on. She had a hypothesis and she tested it out. She considered the violence as a communication to be under-stood, and she listened carefully to the patients as well as to the nurses in a way they had not experienced before. She introduced the idea to them all that not knowing what, or why, and not having an immedi-ate anxiolytic solution was not only acceptable but necessary, in terms of enabling anxieties to surface, be thought about, and contained ther-apeutically.

After turbulent times on the ward, where the pressure she was put under to give in and succumb to the temporarily anaesthetising effect of drugs, the outcome was, to quote from Siobhan,

> Unless a space for reflection is available, many patients who could otherwise benefit from psychological intervention are trapped in regression. This space is provided by the work of the MDT [multidis-ciplinary team]. An interpretive intervention is one where the patients were alerted to a potential external reality of a concerned object. The patients' responses showed a capacity for psychological-mindedness (which had been forgotten by the team, who had, under the enormous pressures they were under, lost theirs) and this psychological mind-edness had been obscured by behaviour (actions and reactions). In a setting with limited resources, a psychoanalytically informed approach proved to have a major therapeutic impact. (O'Connor, 1999, p. 3)

In London, Siobhan became immersed in further work on locked wards, including a focus on female patients, before leading a home treatment team (HTT). Initially, she was Consultant Psychiatrist to two

Southwark-based HTTs, and a couple of years ago these two teams were amalgamated into one, with her as lead. HTTs are the massively important bridge between community mental health teams and in-patient units. They are asked to look after patients with the vast spectrum of psychiatric disorders who become more unwell in the community but can ameliorate with intensive interventions within their homes, even, on rare occasions, up to three times per day, thereby avoiding the disruption to their and their families' lives by an admission to a costly hospital.

Siobhan was always highly professional, a strong and loyal leader, and devoted to bettering the care of the patients. I understand that the team appreciated her generous contribution to their own learning, and her application of psychoanalytic principles within this working environment.

Many of us knew Siobhan from various committees and seminars. She could always be relied upon to give the rest of us presenting a good shake and critique. She could be tough, but she always made one think. I know that Siobhan inspired many junior psychiatrists and clinicians from different disciplines, and she was a great spokesperson for the importance of psychoanalysis in psychiatric settings. She would be the first one to agree that, without her own experience of analysis and the training, she would not have been able to provide such an important and, in our view, essential scaffolding within these psychiatric settings. Siobhan's biggest contribution was reminding psychiatry of its important and essential marriage to psychoanalysis.

How missed she is.

CHAPTER FIVE

Learning from women with psychosis*

Siobhan O'Connor

Introduction

In this chapter, I explore the experience of working as consultant psychiatrist for a psychiatric intensive care unit (PICU) that had been reorganised from a mixed to an all-female unit. I focus on the nature of physical aggression in order to emphasise the clinical challenge for staff working with women suffering from acute and florid psychotic states. Clinical examples are included to illustrate some issues that are of importance for women admitted to hospital.

The analytic literature on women has highlighted the important characteristics that have led to the development of thinking about the maternal transference, aspects of hidden aggression and rivalry, and of secrecy. I suggest that all of these characteristics pose a different challenge for nursing staff in the setting of extreme states of mind and body. In addition, it appeared to me that there has to be a link between

* First published in 2014 in *Psychoanalytic Psychotherapy*, 28(2): 159–75. Copyright © The Association for Psychoanalytic Psychotherapy in the NHS, reprinted by kind permission of Taylor & Francis Ltd, www.tandfonline.com on behalf of The Association for Psychoanalytic Psychotherapy in the NHS.

the countertransference to psychosis and the female-to-female dyad of patient and analyst. I felt that the level of aggression being observed in hospital could not be explained by looking only at the ward and its management problems. If more attention were paid to female development in the provision of treatment for women who have psychotic illnesses, then early management and the care pathway from community to admission might be improved upon.

The clinical setting

With the new millennium, there arrived a series of policy statements from the then government, suggesting that women's distinct mental health needs were going to be met. One of those policies included the removal of mixed sex wards in ninety-five per cent of NHS Trusts by 2002.

The organisation of services within an NHS Trust is that of a public sector corporation headed by a board consisting of executive and non-executive directors. This chapter is about work in an NHS Trust that provides secondary and tertiary mental health care. That is, the Trust is an organisation of hospitals and community services providing mental health treatment and care for the population of four inner city boroughs. The Trust also provides national services in some areas of specialty.

The most recent census shows the population of the four boroughs to be over a million people. Reorganisation into four single-sex PICUs in the Trust had followed that imperative from the Department of Health, which was intended to provide better services for women. Of these four units, one was a twelve-bedded unit for women, located in the hospital of one of the four boroughs. It had been in operation for about three months. I took responsibility for it to help with the transition from a mixed unit to a single sex unit until a permanent consultant was appointed. The other three units were for men, in keeping with the proportions of beds required.

Most of the transfers to the female unit were from acute admission wards. There was a very high proportion of persistent manic or highly aroused psychotic states. The aim of the transfers was to have a brief intervention of two to four weeks during the most disturbed states. Patients transferred to the PICU were those for whom repeated physical intervention had been needed on the acute ward, to restrain the patient or hold her away from others. Other behaviours, such as self-harming, could be managed on acute wards by having extra staff to give more individual attention during crises. Those kept for longer periods on the PICU were a few who were awaiting transfer to alternative longer-stay, high-support or medium secure units. The proportion of patients taken from prison was low, compared with male units. Among the twelve patients at any time we might have had one from prison, but more usually we did not have any. This is a different population to forensic settings: prior to admission, if there had been police intervention following an incident in the community, the police had often used Section 136 of the Mental Health Act (1983) to bring the patient directly to a "place of safety", and charges were not brought. The suite of rooms specifically designed for this purpose was attached to the PICU with access from outside for police and ambulance.

When considering dynamics in a PICU, it is important to appreciate the nature of the medical emergency and why the medical model of illness takes such priority in the minds of doctors and nurses. Organic illness has to be excluded as a diagnosis or a contributory factor in psychotic states. Physical examination is the most basic of investigations required, apart from more intrusive investigations such as blood tests. Any physical intervention on a patient's body requires a therapeutic relationship with some willingness and co-operation by the patient. This may not have been possible on the acute admission ward. There was also the highest level of self-neglect, often due to mental illness, bringing with it the risk of missing co-existent physical illness. Illnesses such as diabetes, more common in mental illness, pose risks to health even if a person has been diligent about diet and medication. During a psychotic episode, lack of attention to diet or diabetic medication led in some to an immediate serious threat to health. Denial of illness during psychosis made the task of identifying physical problems more difficult.

One example was a patient who withdrew to her room, almost mute except for psychotic and angry communication. In the admission ward and following transfer to the PICU, she had refused basic necessities that included her refusal to wash or change her clothes. When she eventually agreed to a bath, the nurses helping her noticed an inflamed toe. As a team, we discussed whether to restrain her to examine her toe, as she had refused examination. She was diabetic and we knew the risks, and therefore made the decision to restrain her. Following examination, while still expressing psychotic ideation, she engaged better in further investigations while accompanied by two nurses on her visits to a general hospital. A specialist in diabetes diagnosed gangrene and was able to discuss with her the planned treatment of amputation of her toe. Her mental state improved almost immediately. She was an intelligent woman who had married, had children, and had worked for many years after her earlier admissions to hospital with schizophrenia. We hypothesised that it was her painful toe and her awareness of the complications of diabetes that had led her into a state of denial with relapse of symptoms of her psychotic illness.

The psychiatric diagnoses of all but a few patients over a year in the unit were of psychotic illnesses, usually within the spectrum of major illnesses of schizophrenia or bipolar affective disorder. One might hypothesise borderline or histrionic personality traits in some patients, but it is common for acute psychoses or affective disorders to present with an exaggeration of personality traits. Cultural background might intensify those traits. Thus, is it clinically unwise to challenge an established diagnosis purely on the basis of current mental state? Abuse of illicit stimulant drugs was relevant in some, but usually as an exacerbating factor in another illness.

My emotional reaction to early observations of the unit

When I started my work in the PICU, it was the heightened disturbance in the staff that was most noticeable to me. It appeared as if the nurses were behaving in a manic way, easily agitated or distracted, and they, in their turn, pressured the doctors with repeated requests. The difficulty in imposing structure with clear boundaries was challenging for the new ward manager and myself. Simple practical measures to tackle the problems took excessive time and negotiation.

One example of opposition to intervention may illustrate. The patients had unsupervised internet access and mobile phones. To any experienced clinician who came new to the ward, such freedom for manic, paranoid, and highly sexualised patients appeared bizarre. Their contact with the outside world increased their own agitation and the pressure upon staff. The patients rang the police, ambulance, or fire services with paranoid delusions. The staff then had to deal with complaints from family, the public, and public emergency services. It made it extremely difficult to assess real concerns. Yet, when we talked of introducing a ban on such easy access, we were met with complaints by patients and many staff that we would be depriving the patients of their human rights. It was as if the nurses were deeply affected to the point of identifying with the patients, without realising that they were doing it. An executive decision made by the ward manager to restrict such access led to immediate improvement.

The agitation that I observed in the nurses was later experienced by me. I experienced the agitation on leaving the unit or on thinking about it outside of work. At times when I felt particularly agitated in my quiet office, I noticed in myself an impulse to return to the nursing station. I think that urge to go back to the nurses might have been a defence, similar to that of the manic patient who was attracted to join the activity on the ward. I think it was an attraction towards projection of my pressure of thoughts into nurses and patients. It may be that the wish was to have some consolation for myself in my usual role as consultant psychiatrist working with the team. This degree of agitation was unusual for me, despite my experience of similar work with acute psychoses where there is a high risk of violence and suicide. In the past, I had managed a mixed PICU for six years, and when I later moved to this Trust, I took responsibility for an acute admission ward in difficulty until we introduced change to help it function better.

Although there have been many changes in mental health services that may account for some differences in this unit, I had never before seen such high agitation or levels of aggressive behaviour in an inpatient setting. I had not previously come across such difficulties in providing medical interventions such as physical examination. The variations between acute wards and PICUs, their physical environment, catchment populations, access to other services within or in addition to the wards in question, all make it difficult to identify what might have been different about this setting. There was a multicultural mix typical of a large inner city. The patients of a PICU are among those often excluded from psychiatric research as too complex and, thus, not typical for any scientific hypotheses. I needed a focus to help me think. I had become accustomed to hearing from staff that all-female units were more difficult but my own experience of all-female units had been before the turn of the century and reduction of beds over the past decade. One of the actions I took when I recognised the pressure on my own capacity to think was to insist upon a reduction in the number of beds being occupied.

Outside of my psychiatric practice within the NHS, which has been in intensive home treatment for many years, I have a private psychoanalytic practice with patients whom I see five days a week. Thus, it was to my analytic mental space that I turned for help to focus upon the overwhelming experience of this unit. I turned to the analytic literature on female development to help me. My first guide was Welldon's book (1988) *Mother, Madonna, Whore*, which I read again. My medical discipline has included a major emphasis on detailed observation as a first step in examination, and Welldon's attention to the way that women use their bodies in communication had particular relevance to the behaviour that I observed.

General observations of behaviour

The aggressive behaviour of women on the ward was recognised to be different from that which was seen as more typical of men. Concerns about vulnerability of women or retaliatory action towards them were more common. Prior to transfer, there was often a history of manic behaviour, in which the patient was invading the space of other patients. There may have been aggressive acts in the community but the emphasis was often on disinhibition in behaviour. In hospital, the behaviours of scratching, biting, and spitting, tearing out a person's hair, accompanied by verbal threats, were more common than in male wards. Nurses said that it was harder to anticipate assaults by women than by men. They reported that signs of bodily arousal were more typically seen in men who were about to attack. They described how men tended to use their bodies to behave in a more overtly threatening manner and to punch or strike. Dilated pupils, clenching of the jaw or fists, and changes in respiration alerted them to possible assaults by men. These signs were usually absent in female patients. There was often a delay between the apparent precipitant and the assault. After assaults, patients often gave their reason for attacking as retaliatory action for something that had occurred earlier.

One example was that of patient N, who said that her sudden assault upon a nurse was because she had not been brought an item the nurse had promised to get from the shop a few days before. In reflection afterwards, staff thought that the incident was linked to the patient's intense feelings about that nurse, but that the immediate trigger was more likely to have been the fact that the nurse had been paying attention to another patient on the ward that day and that N had felt excluded.

In major psychotic illnesses or severe schizophrenic states, smearing of faeces or of bodily fluids may be common to both genders but with the added problem of smearing of menstrual blood by female patients. Now, with the increased incidence and general awareness of blood-borne viruses such as HIV or hepatitis C, biting, scratching, and smearing of blood hold a different meaning for staff and other patients than might have been the case in the past. It is not simply disgust that may be evoked, but fear and risk of serious life-threatening damage. Some patients knowingly threatened staff with their infection, and there were instances when some patients bit or scratched staff when they knew of the possibility of infecting them. This was particularly difficult if patients had to be physically held, an intervention that poses risks for the patient if not expertly done.

Many of our interventions were highly intrusive, necessitated by the nature of the work on a PICU, whether that is to ensure safety, the basic necessities for life and health, or to treat the illness. One frequent form of intrusion is the giving of medication, often taken reluctantly and thus requiring close observation. It may be given by injection against the patient's will. My experience on a mixed intensive care unit had been that, when patients refused medication and were given the alternative of intramuscular injections against their will, they either agreed to take oral medication or agreed after one injection. I had not realised that women would persist in their refusal. In the mixed unit that I had previously managed for six years, I had not encountered a situation when patients persistently refused. This was very disturbing for patients and for staff. Injections given against a patient's will had to be planned ahead, and carried out with extra staff trained in restraint to ensure safety.

In time, I revised my thinking on the difference between men and women with regard to injections. I had previously thought of it only in terms of men's fear of penetration by the needle, for it is such a common observation in general that men fear the needle more than women. When I first became aware of the difference on this unit, I thought it possible that women were more concerned about fear of damage inside their bodies than about the restraint. Behaviours on the ward made me aware of how women appear to be more comfortable with the communication of submission or of apparent submissiveness. In the face of having to take medication that they have refused, they may be relatively less disturbed than men about being held down in restraint. The intervention of restraint may give a masochistic moment of triumph to a woman. However, any assumption that such perverse mechanisms underlie the behaviour of women in acute and florid psychoses underestimates the fluctuation in forms of regressed behaviour. The nature of the therapeutic alliance may change throughout the episode, with fluctuations within hours. These gender differences in behaviour led to an increase in physically intrusive interventions on women when the psychological therapeutic approach would be one that is sensitive to feelings of intrusion, particularly in psychotic illness.

Case example: the theme of pregnancy and contact with children

Delusions of pregnancy were quite common in the psychotic patients admitted to the hospital. Margaret was a twenty-five-year-old mother of two boys, aged eight and three. She was transferred to the unit from an acute ward because of manic behaviour. She was agitated and shouting, but what was most difficult to manage in the acute ward was her intrusiveness towards other patients. This continued through the night when she knocked on their doors while they were sleeping. One of her more persistent delusions was that she was currently pregnant with twins. She exposed her abdomen and rubbed it publicly in the day area. If this was not commented upon, she approached staff tearfully, saying that she was pregnant. She complained that the medication was going to kill her twins. On one occasion, she showed blood on her fingers to nurses. It was blood that she had taken from her vagina while menstruating. She said that her twins were coming out. The nurses therefore had to manage a patient who might spread her blood on to others or themselves. With the risks of HIV or hepatitis so well known, patients usually knew the fear that they evoked. The request for transfer of patients to the PICU focused upon the immediate aggressive acts, but the history of their behaviour often explained more about the difficulty in management and how they evoked emotional reactions. Margaret had been examined and tests done to ensure that she was not pregnant and there was no other cause of vaginal bleeding apart from menstruation. Attention that had to be given to exclude biological change or physical illness distracted from thinking in any depth about another meaning.

One morning, Margaret's mother and aunt arrived with Margaret's three-year-old son Jon to see me. Taking the opportunity, I suggested that Jon could meet his mother. Margaret's mother was reluctant at first, but was eventually persuaded. Margaret was still quite manic in her behaviour on the ward. When Margaret discovered she was going to see her son, she dressed herself well for the visit. She was brought in by a couple of nurses with another standing by just outside of the room. There followed a moving interview in which she hugged her son and talked to him. At times, I had to suggest she was holding him too close, and urged her to relax the pressure. Margaret responded well. Although her speech showed the distractions of the manic illness, she did focus quite well on talking to him. Then, when I started to speak about finishing the interview, her son immediately cried out. It was as if he could predict the nature of my intervention because of the change in tone of my voice. Margaret was in conflict, initially trying to stay to comfort him, but she accepted the urging of the nurses to leave the room. She let her mother and sister comfort him but his cries of protest mounted as she left. A nurse stayed with Jon and his aunt to comfort him and I brought Margaret's mother into another office.

Margaret's mother was apologetic about Jon's behaviour, saying that this would not have happened with his older brother. I talked of his protest and crying as a natural healthy reaction. I said that I thought it was better for Jon to see his mother in the presence of other adults who were caring for her, than to be left with his own imagination about what was happening to his mother in her absence. Margaret's mother went on to say that he was often like this at home, even with her and his aunt. I then realised that her initial reluctance to let Jon see his mother was that his reaction was predictable and that she did not want it to happen.

It was within a few days of this contact that we discussed plans to transfer Margaret back to the admission ward. Her behaviour was calmer; she had not been expressing delusions, and had not mentioned the twins for some time. At the ward round, while we discussed the possibility of transfer, she stroked her abdomen and spoke of her twins. I did not refer directly to her belief in the pregnancy, but said to her that I thought that she was anxious about the future and the planned move to the open ward. Margaret replied, yes, that she was anxious about that. A moment later she added, "Maybe there are no twins, really." Interpretations do not change delusions, and even with recovery they do not completely disappear, it is just that they are not verbalised. I think this was a moment of contact in which she felt her anxieties understood.

The wish for babies held many meanings for the patients. Many of the patients were those who repeatedly got pregnant despite their knowledge that their children had all been taken into care. Margaret was under the care of my home treatment team a couple of years later, with a relapse of her manic illness. By that time, following child protection intervention, her children were legally under the care of her mother. On admission to hospital, patients experienced loss of immediate contact with family and children, and psychotic patients were deprived of their most important attachments, even if their contacts were those into whom they projected persecutory objects. Children do need to be protected from the mothers whose psychoses prevent them from attending to the needs of the children. However, excessive protectiveness in keeping children from seeing their mothers in psychotic states can be misguided. Many of the children had already experienced more of the mother's psychotic state than any other person in her life, and without a third person present. If a child had the opportunity of seeing his mother in the company of adults who were caring for her, we thought that it was more likely to be therapeutic for him too. It seemed, from our limited ability to arrange that contact with their children, that this was also a therapeutic intervention for mothers. In one case, we encouraged the husband of a woman who suffered from a severe puerperal psychosis with catatonic features to bring photos and video film of their newly born baby when he visited her. Our concern was that when she recovered she would not even recognise the baby, who had changed so much in the meantime.

Discussion of gender differences in
psychotic illness and in-patient settings

The consultation document on women's mental health (Department of Health, 2002) addressed the inequalities, discrimination, and disadvantages for women in the delivery of mental health services. McDougall and colleages (2007), in their review of the relevant psychiatric literature, suggested that women appeared to be invisible in biomedical research into schizophrenia. They noted that no dedicated first episode psychosis service existed in their locality (a county in South West England) for people aged more than thirty-five years, yet fifty per cent of women were not diagnosed with schizophrenia until their mid-forties. Research into schizophrenia has shown that there is also a difference in presenting themes. In their symptoms, men are more concerned with political conspiracies and undercover activities and have more grandiose delusions of power, royalty, and divinity. Women typically exhibit far fewer signs of illness: for example they may feel that their body is the wrong shape or they exhibit concern about the way they look. Women also show concerns with romantic preoccupations and false beliefs of pregnancy. Castle and colleagues (2000) suggested that some of the complaints of women were missed because they could be stereotyped as female behaviour. Henri Rey has been quoted in his description of borderline states and the difference between the sexes:

> In the case of women hysterical manifestations, that is to say, hysterical mechanisms of defense mark the underlying personality structure and they show more often than men history on behavior, acting-out, hysterical fits, cunning behavior, and the claustro-agoraphobic syndrome overtly. (Grotstein, 1984, p. 81)

Henri Rey's comment may appear dated, for the term hysterical has almost disappeared from daily use, possibly because of the complaint of stereotyping female behaviour. However, something may have been lost in that attempt to be more scientific and avoid prejudice. In their article on female aggression, Holtzman and Kulish (2003) argue that uniquely feminine characteristics have not been fully recognised or incorporated into psychoanalytic theories. They describe how competitive aggression on the part of young girls, seemingly missing in children's stories and myths, is unconsciously inhibited, disguised, or externalised. In the Greek story of Oedipus, the male's aggression is out in the open. They found that anxiety about separation from the mother was the prominent developmental conflict for girls at the "oedipal" stage, and proposed the term "Persephone complex" from the Greek myth of Persephone. In the myth, Demeter unleashes famine upon the earth following the loss of her daughter, Kore. When her daughter appears again in the story, having been kidnapped and taken to the underworld, she is named Persephone, a change from the innocent child who had been gathering flowers with other girls, into the woman, sexual partner to Hades. Although the myth implies the rape of the daughter by Hades, it also includes her having broken an injunction not to eat in the underworld. She has eaten some seeds of the pomegranate. In the myth, aggression is not visible except in the revengeful retribution of the mother. Aggression does not appear to mark the relationship between Demeter and Persephone. Holtzman and Kulish argue that agency over aggression, like sexuality, is disguised and inhibited in the story as in the female triangular situation itself. They suggest that the myth depicts a frequently occurring defence: that is, the disavowal of agency over sexuality. In their review of the literature, they remark on how little can be found about aggression in women, quoting literature on the general cultural prohibitions against the expression of anger and aggression by girls and women. When aggression is discussed as part of the Oedipus complex situation, it is frequently in the context of female masochism. They suggest that a common thread runs throughout all the writings, the importance to the little girl of preserving her tie to her mother, and the effect of this tie on her expression and handling of aggression.

The power of secrets and disguise by women is discussed further in the analytic literature. Welldon (1988), in her work on perversions in women, noted the importance of the body in the little girl's development. The womb and capacity to have babies is an inner possession of power. She wrote of the female use of the whole body as sexual object rather than the phallo-centrism seen in male perversions. Balsam (1996) wrote that within the woman's body lies the secret of giving life and the potential to produce an actual baby. In her article on secrets, Kulish (2002) wrote of the establishment of a sense of separation from the mother and why women especially treasure secrets. She writes about inner possessions and how the first lie breaks the tyranny of parental omniscience. She described secrecy, one weapon of the power of the weak, as a resource left to women. With this power of secrets in mind, the adjective "cunning" used by Henri Rey may hint at something in the dynamic that includes a different experience of assaults that are hidden or unexpected.

Freud identified surprise as a pre-condition of traumatic reaction (Freud, 1920g). In the unit, the assaults had that character of surprise for the person assaulted. They may have appeared as if secretly planned if the presence of psychotic thought processes were not taken into account. I did not think of the behaviours of sudden assaults as arising in the context of conscious secretive planning, but as of sudden impulsive action arising in the context of paranoid ruminations. I believed that an impulsive bodily communication was enacted when words were not experienced by a patient as a powerful enough communication. That was generally in keeping with the view of the nurses, who would have had no difficulty in expressing an alternative view if a diagnosis of personality disorder was considered by them to be more appropriate. In contrast, the more typical behaviour of a male patient was that of an intimidating posture as a display of power or intimidation, followed by an assault.

Some of the high level of disturbance in the PICU was in keeping with changes observed generally following reduction in beds in mental health service provision (Lodge, 2012). Since the earliest work on the dynamics of in-patient settings, many of the dynamics have been discussed in mixed and in single-gender units (Menzies Lyth, 1988a; Stanton & Schwartz, 1954). Consultation and reflective practice within institutions is now a major contribution by psychoanalysts. More recently, since the loss of the larger asylums, with reduced numbers of admission beds in this country, the overall raised level of disturbance in the hospitals has been described from a psychodynamic perspective (Chiesa, 1993; Fagin, 2001).

The fact that this was a newly developed ward of the twenty-first century, with a new team working together, might have been seen as the main problem that led to the disturbance in staff. Nevertheless, in the two years since my work on this ward, the Trust's centrally collected data on aggression and violence has still noted that the level of violence is higher on the female intensive care unit than in the male units. However, it is very hard to validate any figures regarding aggression on the wards. Arguments are made that one ward is better at recording than another, or doubt is cast over the severity of injuries sustained in violent acts. If research is to be valid, then gender differences need to be considered in looking at the data.

Emotional reactions of staff, whether as a function of the ward setting, or as a function of reaction to individual patients, are all important in the activity of recording data. Defence mechanisms lead to surges of recording of minor incidents that at other times are tolerated to excess. Thus, it is relevant to consider whether there is any gender difference in the countertransference with female patients or in the dynamic between females kept confined in a locked setting.

The nursing role is often considered maternal, whether nurses are male or female (Fabricius, 1995), and there are more female nurses on a single-sex unit. The relationship between female analysts and female patients as described by Kulish and Holtzman (2003) has appeared in keeping with some observations. They write that the beneficial effects of the countertransference in this dyad are frequently stressed in psychoanalytic literature. On the more negative side, however, celebration of the beneficial effects of reworking of separation themes between women may obscure other issues. Female analysts often miss, or misinterpret, "oedipal" (and/or paternal) transferences. Kulish and Holtzman (2003) quote many writers who describe female analysts responding defensively to the competition and envy of their female patients and often resist being seen as the rival "oedipal" mother. Instead, they tend to get involved or lost in earlier, pre-oedipal mother–daughter issues and often become too merged or over-identified with their patients. They write of female analysts becoming "too maternal" and overprotective. Might some of these characteristics of the dyad be applied to the tendency of staff in psychiatry to see the patients' behaviour as due to their psychosis, or secondary to earlier traumas in their lives, seeing the patient as victim of trauma, rather than seeing a female aspect of character?

Rosenfeld describes the acting out of a psychotic patient in regression as "a desperate attempt to induce the analyst to act out towards the patient with over friendly behaviour . . ." (Rosenfeld, 1965, p. 206). He said that when there was excessive acting out, the danger was that the patient might suddenly give up most of his ego activities and his relations to objects in everyday life, and show regressive behaviour in the analysis, acting like a small dependent child. This seems to be a very good description of what happens in in-patient wards. Rosenfeld's description of the pressure on the analyst to respond in a friendly manner, rather than interpret the negative transference, is important in general psychiatry.

This may be exacerbated with female staff working with female patients. I was prompted to think about the young age range of nurses while I watched a couple of young female student nurses in the day room standing close together. They were talking to each other while some older patients had turned up the music and were dancing around the room in a manic way, something that was likely to lead to aggressive outbursts. It appeared to me as if the student nurses were protecting each other by excluding the activity from their minds. I thought of what their presence would mean to some of these patients and how envy of these attractive girls, their apparent success, and future prospects might even fuel the loud demonstration of manic behaviour as a kind of protest, or maybe even to provoke fear in the nurses. I also thought that the presence of men to whom these patients could relate as peers may have had beneficial aspects in mixed wards that had not been considered when thinking about the protection of women.

Case example: physical containment of manic states

The following example is quite typical of ward rounds and of dynamics on the ward. Beatrice, a thirty-eight-year-old woman who suffered from a manic illness, came to the ward round. Her new community social worker had joined us and this was to be her first meeting with the patient. Beatrice entered the room with what appeared a dignified and slightly superior air. When she sat down, she looked around her and interrupted my attempt at an introduction to the process by starting to speak as if she were conducting interviews. She asked the senior nurse about sanitary towel provision on the ward. She held up a large incontinence pad that looked as big as a nappy and said that this was what she had been given. The nurse explained that the ward did not provide sanitary towels and asked how she had got the pad. The display of the pad was effective in providing a shocking image of a patient being humiliated by inadequacies of resources on the ward. It was a false picture of conditions on the ward, but it made its impact over any discussion that followed. The patient was dismissive of the nurse's answer. She turned her attention to other members of staff present, with other complaints that might have sounded rational to a person naïve to the setting. The junior doctor, for example, was quizzed on blood tests with what appeared an implied complaint that Beatrice was not being given appropriate information. Sometimes, staff said in their answers that they had addressed the complaint, or they corrected her impressions, but each faced argument and then dismissal by her as she turned to the next person.

When Beatrice allowed herself to be introduced to her social worker, she started by forcibly asking questions about access to her children. She insisted on getting an answer as to what service the social worker was going to provide for her, interrupting with new questions when an attempt was made to respond. The questions were in denial of the reality of her situation. Her access had been refused before admission because of her neglect of her children and concerns about their safety when they were with her. The discussion appeared to me like an examination by Beatrice of how much the social worker knew of the complexity of the ongoing legal processes. As the questioning by Beatrice became increasingly hostile and obviously out of touch, I intervened with authority, saying that enough had been said and that she could explore these questions later.

I started to encourage Beatrice to leave the ward round. Following an exchange that might have appeared calm or measured, albeit out of touch, she turned her focus towards me. There was no sign that she would accept that she had to leave. The nurses stood up to encourage her, but eventually had to escort her out, physically holding her.

Beatrice was transferred back to an acute ward about a week after this ward round, having been in the PICU for three weeks. It was a different acute ward than the one from which she had previously been transferred. Over the next two weeks she was given increasing leave from the acute ward with a view to discharge. She was then transferred back to the PICU, after having become quite manic and violent in behaviour again. The re-admission to the intensive care unit was for another three weeks. In the intensive care unit, she dominated the group and roused other patients to fight with each other. She did this while appearing calm and apparently rational and sophisticated. She told one patient, for example, that another patient had made vicious or defamatory comments about her. She chose her subject, picking one who looked up to her and was known to be quicker to act. A violent episode then occurred between two other patients. Beatrice made disapproving remarks to the nurses or doctors about other patients fighting, as if she were an observer.

Following the second transfer, we were more specific in our physical intervention. In the company of a nurse, Beatrice stayed apart, in a quiet area away from other patients, except at mealtimes. This could be managed by one nurse but only with others nearby, ready to intervene physically, if necessary. This was similar to the ward round where the nurses calmly showed their strength together as a team. With a manic patient, there was quite a persistent need of verbal communication from the nurse to keep the patient calm and co-operating so that physical interventions were not required. Beatrice accepted this intervention although, with her pressure of activity and speech, she tended to be drawn towards the activity in the ward.

The ward round was a setting in which the team worked together to contain the patient. The display of the incontinence pad, followed by questions focused upon each professional, appeared to be an intense focus upon failures by each professional. She did not say anything that acknowledged her paranoid ideation, or her grandiose delusions in the way that a psychiatric interview would elicit, but her actions and words were in the nature of demands for responses. She appeared to portray herself as the concerned mother deprived of seeing her children. Her verbal provocation was such that she mocked or denigrated others, but with a demand for a response that could not reassure her. The alternative response, one of aggression, was more freely available to her on a ward with patients who would act upon provocation. In her grandiose delusions, she believed that she was superior, with many talents, and her persecutors in the ward were the doctors and nurses who were detaining her. Such delusions were present in some interviews but usually demonstrated by speech as action, such as mockery or denigration, rather than verbalised in the content of her speech.

Beatrice's case illustrates the nature of pressurised speech, which may be persistent in manic states. In the presence of the full team, part of her difficulty in sustaining a conversation was shown by her attention moving from one person to the next. Sustained physical restraint was not needed for containment, but just enough strength and firmness so that she knew that we did have the physical power to hold her. A communicative approach by nurses on the ward required constant individual attention, which included monitoring her level of arousal.

In the presence of other aroused patients, it was less obvious that she was aroused. In an acute ward that did not have these resources for individual attention, the level of arousal increased until an assault occurred.

Further thoughts on countertransference

I have described the nature of the medical emergency of the PICU and why examination and medical investigations are so important. If one cannot focus upon the complex medical problems, the risks are high, and that was my main concern when I asked for a reduction in beds for a period. Since I first worked in a mixed intensive care unit, I also realised that the threat of physical injury to staff or other patients takes precedence over other countertransference reactions.

Although the nurses have always been interested in the dynamics or meaning of symptoms that I discussed with them, I soon found that it did not appear to make a difference in the way that they reported clinical material to me. In contrast to other acute mental health settings, it appeared at times as if they suddenly dropped interest in our more thoughtful discussions. Following my own reflection on this, I suggested in an earlier article that nurses have to maintain the attitude of a vigilant mother with her child. The mother ensures that the environment is safe and apparently allows freedom of movement until she is alerted to danger. She then intervenes to neutralise, taking the child away from the danger, or stopping its activity (O'Connor, 1999). In the case of nurses with their patients, it is not only the safety of the patients that is important. They have to be attentive enough to their own safety. The experience of injury to a nurse affects more than the individual. For her colleagues, this goes further than empathy and identification, for it has real effects on the functioning of the team. Injury that limits a nurse in her ability, or leads to sick leave, affects that individual as well as the team's ability to function with overtime or with temporary staff.

The psychoanalytic literature on borderline psychoses, or dynamics in which manic defences are productive of countertransference responses, tends to underestimate the importance of the physical threat in this setting. The available literature on psychotic processes is more relevant in a ward setting, where there is time and space to have an engagement that is not focused primarily on physical safety. In the intensive care unit, the experience of engagement in verbal communication is a welcome relief for nurses who choose to work in areas of acute psychoses. As soon as safety is ensured, plans are made to transfer the patient back to another ward.

The response by an experienced psychoanalyst who read my first draft of this chapter was to say that there was too much violence in it. I realised that I had intentionally included clinical accounts that might alert the reader to the experience of working in a PICU. The problem with that was that my descriptive account had become an attack on the reader, which is in keeping with the more common reaction to the unit, in which staff of any discipline tend to stay away, or make only brief visits, with few visiting to work with those who might engage long enough to make occasional sessions viable. If the threat of violence is such that injuries are still occurring regularly, it may be demoralising to staff to focus too much on their emotional reactions, as if jt the problem is due to something internal, such as the functioning of their team. I think that may lead to the defensiveness shown when attention is drawn to the level of violence in the ward.

In a ward where bodily communication was the main reason for transfer, Bion's description is relevant: "Language is employed by the schizophrenic in three ways; as a mode of action, as a method of communication, and as a mode of thought" (Bion, 1967, p. 24). If the speech of patients is not heard and communication with staff does not reassure the patient of there being a meaningful response or containment, then physical action by the patient may be the next form of communication. On the ward, the task for the nurses was to monitor communication in such a way that they picked up on intensity and pressure of speech, as well as bodily communication. The actions of a patient such as Margaret, walking around rubbing her abdomen, would be something that would be noticed by the nurses as evidence of activity of her delusional state. Sensitivity to these forms of communication also required attention to details such as how the patients related to each other. In Beatrice's case, this required strength and firmness in physical interventions. Observation and attention to these details is a different task to that of other therapeutic settings where verbal engagement is the priority. The need to act with strength in a calm way has to be combined with that sensitivity to all modes of communication.

Beyond the need for firm structure, there were aspects to the behaviour of women that may have evoked different emotional reactions. Secretiveness, the hidden nature of aggression, scratching and biting, all evoke different reactions. Smearing is an act of protest that may appear designed to elicit a response in the stronger object, whether that is of retaliation or of retreat. I thought most powerful was the ease with which women would use an appearance of submission to avoid conflict. This was in keeping with Rosenfeld's description of regressive acting out.

In the face of stronger persecutory objects, women may find it easier to show apparent submission. In the countertransference, the adjectives "cunning" and "hysterical" may convey something of the attitude of the person who has detected the agency of aggression hidden in those acts of submission. It can be difficult for any professional to face patients who plead, express disappointment, or look dejected, when their requests for freedom are refused. More overt acts of aggression, which are more typical of men, are somewhat easier to understand and to prepare for. It was more often the case with women than with men that their vulnerability was highlighted in risk assessments before discharge, along with the history of aggressive acts. In this, there is a link to the dynamic in domestic violence where it is women who are most often assaulted (Dwyer, 1995).

The care pathway for women from community to intensive care

It has been argued that, because psychiatric beds are rationed, this rationing will mean that young men with behaviours that bring them to the notice of the psychiatric services owing to their perceived dangerousness will be more likely to be admitted and treated. Women, it is suggested, who might have similar levels of a psychiatric disorder but who may not appear so dangerous, will be less likely to receive treatment (Payne, 1995). The different forms of communication by women with hidden aspects or secrets may contribute to missing early symptoms. Apart from those patients of either gender who might be violent in action for other reasons, the aggressive behaviour seen in manic or floridly psychotic patients is often only seen during the most severe state of their psychosis. Following admission, the setting of an environment in which women are held together in a confined space is common to medium-secure and intensive psychiatric units. In acute psychiatry, however, the repetition of transfers between services before and after admission to hospital is due to difficulties in containment in acute psychotic states. Transfers during the acute episode may exacerbate the psychotic state. An increased frequency of transfer occurs in a care pathway in which containment cannot be provided in a local ward. This experience may also be the case for those men who have been transferred from one borough to another, but transfers are more common for women as fewer inpatient beds are needed for women. This has led to the fact that women have more transfers in the pathway to the one specialised PICU.

There may also be greater sensitivity in woman to loss in relationships. Relationships have been described as more important for women in their development than power or potency, which is more important for men. Chodorow (1978) and Lerner (1980) have suggested that separation is especially difficult and salient for the little girl as compared with the little boy. Holtzman and Kulish (2000) argued that the anxieties of separation from mother, particularly in the context of pre-oedipal troubled relationships, were of greater importance than power or powerlessness as illustrated in the Oedipus complex. In adults with psychotic illness, both genders experience loss and separation, but it appears ironic that women whose psychotic illnesses suggest the highest incidence of disturbed pre-oedipal object relationships are exposed to repeated transfers in specialised services. A bio-medical approach that places less importance on the therapeutic relationship as an agent for change may be exacerbating the illness in those for whom that relationship is providing a special service.

PART II

STAFF AND ORGANISATIONAL
NEEDS AND CHALLENGES

CHAPTER SIX

Reflective psychiatry: psychoanalytic theory in everyday clinical practice

Turlough Mills and Mike Smith

Introduction

This chapter is written from the perspective of two psychiatrists, who are both new consultants: one working with children and adolescents in the NHS and one working with adults in forensic secure services in the private sector. They have both been taught psychoanalytic thinking during their specialist and sub-specialist training and have both been in personal therapy.

In this introduction it may be useful to consider the following questions: why should psychoanalytic thinking be considered useful for practising psychiatrists? What is meant by psychoanalytic thinking?

As psychiatrists, we are clear that our clinical practice draws extensively on psychoanalytic understanding and experience and that, without this psychoanalytic perspective, we could not function as effectively as we do. It is our belief that our ability to think psychoanalytically conveys humanity—a fundamental recognition that all patients are, like their psychiatrists, complex human beings, and that the relationship between the patient and the professional constitutes the most valuable resource in rendering clinical practice and help meaningful.

Psychoanalytic thinking proposes the existence of an unconscious mind. This is the repository for all lived experience, including very early conflicts between our instinctual urges and inhibitory processes. Freud described the most basic instincts as Eros, towards life, and Thanatos, towards death, and further suggested that such urges, left unchecked, must lead to ruination for both society and the individual (Freud, 1920g). Therefore, he suggested a number of mechanisms for the inhibition of such urges: for example, the internalising of parental authority.

Taken together, these unconscious conflicts between urge and inhibition are described as phantasies. Phantasies exist outside of conscious awareness but exert influence upon the individual. A core tenet of psychoanalysis might be that the patient (and by extension all human beings) exists in a continuously dynamic relationship to his unconscious phantasies, and that this manifests in daily situations involving love, hatred, and indifference, all occurring without conscious awareness. A psychoanalytic treatment might aim to help the patient see how his present behaviour and thinking are products of his unconscious phantasy life. We suggest that such insights—by definition unreachable through self-introspection alone—lead to a richer lived experience.

Psychoanalytic treatments and thinking are not currently "fashionable" within the provision of mental health services. Compared to the forced simplicity of cognitive–behavioural models of the mind, with their associated promises of rapid psychic change following minimal intervention, Freudian ideas might seem unnecessarily complex, and even fantastic.

However, to us, evidence of phantasy and of the unconscious mind can be seen in the everyday clinical practice of psychiatric work. As psychiatrists, we do not view patients as empty vessels holding mental illness, which can be worked upon in a hermetically sealed world, free from the contamination of disturbing feelings, joyful feelings, or the suffering caused by an inability to feel. Patients, like their psychiatrists, are complicated individuals, full of wishes, fears, dreads, and irrationality. Thus, when the patient and psychiatrist meet, there is a conscious clinical interaction, wherein the psychiatrist asks the patient about her condition, is answered, and acts upon that, and there is another interaction taking place simultaneously and unconsciously. By definition, neither patient nor psychiatrist knows what is happening in their unconscious minds, but they can trace the evidence of unconscious influences there and then, or afterwards, through what they say, what they do, how they feel and behave, and what they do not say, do not do, and do not feel. Hence, the importance of the title of this chapter: "Reflective psychiatry". The work of reflection, in our view, is equally as important as the work of communicating with the patient.

There is, of course, no such thing as a straightforward patient, any more than there is such a thing as a straightforward person. However, there might be a tendency for psychiatrists to think in terms of straightforward patients or not straightforward patients. The (conscious) fantasy of the straightforward patient is of one who receives her treatment (gratefully) and gets better—that is, offers no resistance to the help offered. Even were such patients to exist, it is our experience that, as consultant psychiatrists in our particular specialties, we are not asked to see them. Rather, we are called upon to see those who resist their cure. We are asked to see the patients who are stuck, those for whom nothing else (or no one else) has "worked". These patients tend to be risky and frightening; they often arrive on our therapeutic doorsteps carrying a narrative of burn-out—a form of professional dissociation—within the people and systems that have tried to hold them.

One characteristic of this group of patients is that they do not do as they are told. They are not "good" patients. They do not get better when they should. They relate to those linked to them in professional capacities in powerful and often unsettling ways. They might appear to hate and love their psychiatrists in unequal and varying doses. They might defy the potency of the psychiatrist or, conversely, become impotent and subservient to them. They might invite the professional to abuse them, or to reject them, and they might get under their skin in a hundred different ways. They might sabotage their therapies or their treatments in ways that appear chronically and profoundly baffling and frustrating.

These patients will frequently have "attracted" a diagnosis of some variant of a personality disorder and have often had experience of significant early emotional deprivation and trauma, including physical or sexual abuse, often at the hands of primary carers. They could be considered as people who have been failed, who then evoke feelings of failure in professionals. Their capacity to form meaningful and trusting relationships with others is impaired. They appear to live in a world full of threat and existential dread. They will often have multiple contacts with multiple professionals and in those relationships will often repeat, in their interactions, the cycles of a toxic form of dependency, rejection, and abandonment, which they have internalised within themselves. The invitation to professionals to join in these disturbing relationships is extended unconsciously through projection and unconscious reminders evoked in the professional of their own areas of disturbance. All involved can end up reinforcing maladaptive and destructive patterns of behaviour. This is likely to leave both patients and professionals feeling hopeless and despairing.

Psychiatrists have a particular part to play in these situations, as they can offer an observational perspective, both in their relationship with the patient and as witnessing the relationships between the patient and other professionals in a team. They could be well placed to offer a triangulated position, employing their familiarity with a system of thought, which recognises the role of the unconscious in relationships, as a means of disentangling the complicated feelings that surround difficult patients.

This chapter shows how these psychiatrists use their recognition of a shared humanity, in which both patient and professional are equally susceptible to emotional urges and psychic conflict. Four clinical vignettes with associated discussion attempt to illustrate how psychoanalytic thinking complements psychiatric practice. In addition, these vignettes relate to four different clinical domains, which pose specific challenges and are likely to be familiar to all psychiatrists. The domains chosen are:

1. Phenomenology and diagnosis: how an understanding of countertransference can help make sense of a problematic presentation.
2. Managing suicide risk in the adolescent population: the role of the psychiatrist in containing anxiety.
3. Keeping hold of "bothersome" patients: recognising how troubling patients can pass through the system—both the service and the mind of the professional—without touching the emotional sides.
4. Fear in the workplace: guarding against professional sadism.

Emotional phenomena and phenomenology

A junior doctor attended the paediatric ward to complete an emergency assessment on a patient with a history of childhood sexual abuse at the hands of a relative. The patient was reported to have been in great distress at admission. When the doctor arrived, the patient was calmly watching a comedy show on television and finishing a second helping of pudding. She was being attentively looked after by a ward nurse. On seeing the doctor, the patient appeared to become agitated and described a fearsome hallucinated figure in the corner of the room urging her to harm herself and others. The patient described herself as dangerously mad and begged for an effective intervention from the doctor. She asked for medication to "knock her out" or to be "locked up somewhere safe". The nurses on the ward joined the patient in her requests.

The doctor felt frustrated and angry. In supervision after the encounter, she described the nurses as "in league" with the patient and unconsciously colluding with a "false" presentation. She felt "over a barrel", unable to believe the patient's account of her internal experience, yet frightened of what she might do. She felt tyrannised by what she perceived to be a deception.

This kind of experience may be familiar to all psychiatrists, and is likely to have been encountered many times throughout their training and, indeed, into their consultant careers. The patient unconsciously wounds the doctor's competence—undermines her professional potency and her sense of fairness, to the extent that her ability to act helpfully might be jeopardised. The doctor might feel resentful that she has been "tricked" by the patient, souring her desire to help. The feeling of helplessness might no longer be located only in the patient, or not in the patient at all; it is the doctor who feels helpless. In such a situation, if the doctor has no concept of an unconscious mind, she has no recourse other than to assume a conscious mind is lying.

One of the earliest skills that all doctors must learn is how to ask the "right questions" of their patients. This art—of knowing what the "right questions" might be—refers to éliciting information that helps to formulate a diagnosis to assist meaningful and evidence-based management, or even a cure, and is referred to within the medical profession as taking a history. Medical and surgical doctors might ask their patients where their pain is located, when it began, whether it fluctuates, and whether anything either exacerbates or relieves it. The story they elicit gives an idea of what might be causing the symptoms and directs them to appropriate examination and investigation.

This medical paradigm is used by psychiatrists, although it does not map quite as neatly on to the country of the mind as it does the contours of the body in physical medicine. The psychiatric doctor in training is also taught to "take a history", asking questions about mood, sleep, appetite, perceptual disturbance, and ideas and thoughts. Knowing what the "right questions" might be is not predicated only on "discovering" the diagnosis, but on moving beyond the diagnosis of the *problem* to an attempt to meet and to build a relationship with the *person* who presents in a state of mental disturbance, mental pain, or an absence, or emptiness, which is filled with the paranoia of a persecuting presence. The psychiatrist must also ask questions about the patient's family, childhood, development, social relationships, and recreational activities. This history, together with her observations of the patient, is then used to make her provisional and differential diagnoses. Differential and provisional diagnoses are used to inform further investigation and treatment.

Investigation of the mind might indeed involve brain scans or blood tests, but it also usually involves waiting, talking, listening, and spending time getting to know the person. A patient who describes feeling consistently sad with no obvious reason, who finds himself unable to do what he used to do, who has lost pleasure in life, and who presents as withdrawn and slowed in the assessment, might be diagnosed with depression and prescribed psychoactive medication or a talking therapy, or both. Sometimes, if the risk is deemed too great, they might be offered an admission to hospital, on a voluntary or, sometimes, an involuntary basis.

The art of the history-taking and the observational mental state assessment are largely unchanged from when they were described in the eighteenth century by psychiatrists such as Emil Kraeplin and Kurt Shneider and the philosopher Karl Jaspers. Some of the diagnostic categories might have shifted and some causal associations between phenomenology and diagnosis might have weakened, but modern psychiatry still places history-taking and observational assessment at its heart.

Most psychiatrists, ourselves included, would see the above as scientific endeavour. That is, developing a hypothesis about what is happening in the mind of the patient and then testing this hypothesis, prepared to refute one's view of a patient and learn from the evidence that the null hypothesis is confirmed and a different view, yet to be discovered, is more likely to be right. Asking questions, allowing the patient to tell his story, and observing how he does it can give a good insight into the inner life of the patient. However, it is also our opinion that such an insight must be informed by the feelings of the doctor when he is with the patient, which can be considered to be in part an emotional reaction to the patient.

Freud named this emotional reaction to the patient countertransference, and this has become one of the few psychoanalytic terms that is readily used throughout psychiatry, interestingly more so than transference, or the emotional response of the patient to the doctor, which Freud considered to be of central therapeutic importance (Freud, 1910d). Sometimes, a psychiatrist can identify and understand that when he feels, for example, sad or brought down, these feelings might relate to the mind of his patient. If he can recognise the link between his feelings and the potential feelings of his patient, this can further validate both the patient's history of being miserable for a long time and the doctor's observations of a patient who sits slumped in their chair unable to meet the doctor's eyes. The doctor feels with the patient, rather than solely observing the feelings of the patient—the basis of empathy. However, there are a great many patients where the triad of history, observation, and countertransference do not hang together. In fact, it is our experience of our own specialities that such patients might even make up the majority of those that we see.

Of particular interest are those patients who describe "serious" psychopathology, such as hallucinations or suicidality, yet who fail to "convince" the doctor of the emotional reality or genuineness of their described symptoms. It should be noted that we are not describing patients who present with grossly incongruous affect—that is, patients who might laugh when they should be sad, as can be observed in some psychotic illnesses, or who appear emotionally deadened, as can often present in depression—but, rather, a category of patients who seek to convince the doctor that they are suffering from some specific pathology, which the doctor believes that they are not.

One understandable response to such a patient, from a doctor trained to match history with observation and to refer to her own countertransference for a validation of that match, is to conclude that she is being defrauded and deceived when her emotional response does not validate the patient's description of symptoms. This concrete approach maps well on to physical medicine, but not on to psychological medicine. It can lead doctors (and other professionals) to an automatic process of sorting out their patients into opposite categories of "genuine" or "fraudulent". "Genuine" patients are those who are perceived to have a "true mental illness", which they can describe accurately and convincingly to the doctor, and who can be observed as suffering appropriate symptoms (and, importantly, to be suffering symptoms that can be treated successfully), so that the doctor feels in an ego-syntonic and potent state of mind: a good doctor with a good patient. "Fraudulent" patients, on the other hand, are felt to be making up symptoms of an illness that they do not have in an attempt to fool those around them—the bad patient who has made the doctor feel bad.

In the case above, the doctor felt deceived by her patient. The descriptions of the hallucinations did not fit with her initial impressions of a normal woman enjoying television, food, and the attentions of a nurse. She also felt alienated and under attack by the nurse. In this situation, the "true needs" of the patient remained obscure, occluded by the doctor's resentment. The doctor, unable to understand how she was being used unconsciously, was, thereby, rendered powerless to help—the pained recipient of feelings of exclusion and powerlessness. The doctor was in an unconscious identification with the patient.

Patients who "behave like this" often "attract" the unattractive diagnosis of personality disorder (in America, borderline personality disorder, in the UK, emotionally unstable personality disorder). As personality is considered to be fluid until the age of eighteen, such patterns of behaviour observed in the under-eighteen population (adolescence) may be described as "emerging" personality disorder— there is uncertainty as to whether this might be normal adolescent fluidity in a developing identity. Personality disorders are considered to be developmental conditions, which arise in infancy and early childhood, going "underground" in latency, and then resurfacing in adolescence and persisting as a stable pattern of developmental difficulty into adulthood. Personality disorders are characterised by severe disturbances in relationships, intrapersonally, in the person, and interpersonally, as manifest in attitude and behaviour. They cause great distress to the sufferer and have a marked impact on social functioning: that is, a marked and damaging impact on the capacity to form and sustain fulfilling and creative relationships in love and work.

The aetiology of personality disorder attracts a range of theoretical opinion, but there appears to be a strong correlation with emotional deficit and adverse, often cumulative, traumatic events in childhood. There is an especially strong link between persistent emotional invalidation of the child by the carer and development of the disorder. Sexual abuse—which can be thought of as emotional invalidation of the most destructive kind—correlates very highly with the diagnosis.

Children who have consistently met with unpredictable, confusing, and frightening responses to their emotional needs from their carers are likely to develop into adults who are pathologically unable to seek out and reciprocate to healthy care. They are likely to express their needs and manage their emotions in ways that might appear deeply unhelpful to those around them.

In the vignette introduced above, the junior doctor felt unable to find a "way in" to make meaningful emotional contact with the patient. The discrepancy between the patient's reported symptoms and the doctor's own observations obscured a true emotional understanding of the patient's internal state. The doctor developed a rapid bias and became "stuck on" the patient's apparent falseness. She found herself reacting to that assumption, rather than being able to recognise her feelings of resentment, exclusion, and impotence as representing an emotional state, which the patient needed to have understood.

Feeling excluded by the apparent alliance between nurse and patient, the doctor felt that her competence was being undermined by a fellow professional. In psychoanalytic theory, this represents an oedipal exclusion, the doctor being unconsciously placed in the position of being the outsider looking on and seeing a couple in infuriating, enraging, comfortable togetherness. Although she regarded herself as a good and experienced clinician, during the assessment she found herself feeling useless and foolish. She was, however, able to recognise her inner disturbance and reflect on it internally. In supervision, she was able to reflect that her "stuck" feelings might have arisen from the interplay of the relationships between her, the patient, and the nurse, rather than being located only in her. She wondered whether the alienating "falseness" of the encounter was an indication that something was being hidden in the situation, in the patient, or in herself. The patient's true vulnerability appeared to be masked by agitation and the dramatic account of anxiety-provoking hallucinations. The doctor began to feel that the psychopathological situation was the one that she had first observed, with the patient and the nurse "stuck" together, leaving her feeling pushed out and impotent.

She described to the patient that she felt herself being kept away from something important and wondered aloud whether the patient was very frightened of losing care and being left out in the cold. These interventions appeared to allow the patient to speak in a more "real" way about her anxieties should she be discharged from the ward and the worry of limitations in any follow-up care. This intervention for the patient was heard by the nurse and appeared to allow her, in turn, to relinquish her over-protective role and return to her normal duties.

In this case, the doctor's examination of her own feelings enabled her to make sense of a situation that she had been experiencing as opaque. By naming her stuckness to herself and then wondering aloud about the possible echo of this experience for the patient, she was able to achieve some movement in the assessment and make a contact with the patient's fearful and powerless inner state. Together, they were able to formulate a safe discharge plan and the patient managed to leave the ward and, thereby, managed an experience of being excluded, which she had defended against by unconsciously locating the problem of exclusion in the doctor.

Suicide risk in the adolescent population: resisting admission

The doctor assesses a boy for an emergency presentation. The previous night he had absconded from the residential unit where he had recently been placed, and took a small overdose of an over-the-counter cough preparation, with the expressed intention of killing himself. He has a number of failed placements in his history of care.

The boy is pleasant and engages well with the assessment. He talks positively about his current placement and describes himself as happy there. He states that he is no longer suicidal but acknowledges that he has a long history of harming himself while in a suicidal state of mind.

Outside the assessment suite, the doctor meets with the social worker and a representative of the police. Both of them are frightened and very anxious. They want an immediate and intensive therapy to be delivered from the local Child and Adolescent Mental Health Services.

Failing that, they want the patient to be admitted to a psychiatric hospital for treatment of his mental illness.

This section discusses the assessment and management of suicide risk, especially in relation to in-patient admissions to manage risk. It should be noted that the themes relating to suicide risk are different from those involving risk to others.

Assessment and management of the risk that the patient poses to himself and to others is an area in which the psychiatrist is required to be expert. All mental health professionals assess and manage risk with their patients on a day-to-day basis. However, with complex presentations, they are likely to turn to a psychiatric opinion to assist with this.

With regard to suicidality, there is a recognised spectrum, from fleeting suicidal ideas to completed suicide. Most individuals with suicidal ideas do not go on to complete suicide. However, many will go on to deliberately harm themselves, using various methods, including cutting themselves, using ligatures, and taking overdoses of medication. Individuals who harm themselves are at a higher risk of suicide and death through misadventure.

One possible response to those patients who present themselves as suicidal is to arrange an admission to a psychiatric hospital. The purpose of an admission would be to assess mental state and initiate appropriate treatment and would be considered when the risk posed by the patient is judged too great to be contained safely in the community. Carers and patients might often request that this is considered as a first response, rather than as a last resort. Children who present in suicidal states of mind cause considerable concern, and the idea that they should be looked after within the community setting can be highly anxiety provoking.

Practically speaking, there are far fewer beds available as a national resource than there are patients who could be admitted to them. Generic child and adolescent beds number in the hundreds, young people in significant crisis number in the thousands. It is not feasible with this infrastructure to admit all young people who present as high risk to themselves. More importantly, it is not clinically desirable.

In-patient admissions are sometimes necessary when all community resources have been exhausted. This includes the capacity of the family or other carers to cope with the emotional demands of the young person. However, the benefit of any admission must be weighed against any potential risks.

In-patient environments offer a degree of physical security. Patients are contained within a building, their activities can be restricted, and they can be placed under observation. Generic units are not locked environments, but patients can be physically prevented from leaving through application of the appropriate Mental Health Act. Patients should be able to access structured therapies, for example, individual psychology, child psychotherapy, family therapy, and behavioural activities. They should also have access to group therapies where they can learn along with, and from the experiences of, their peers. Most importantly—or perhaps most differently from what can be provided within the community—they can have access to the continuous therapeutic care provided by psychiatric nurses and healthcare support workers.

Each of these beneficial aspects of an in-patient admission has a potentially destructive association and it is possible for the patient's condition to worsen over the course of the admission, as a result of the admission itself. For example, admitted patients, especially those who have some deficiencies in their own experience of caring, might become overly dependent on the therapeutic environment, where a compassionate listener can be found at all hours of the day and night. This can make the prospect of discharge appear insurmountably painful and to be resisted. Additionally, while healthy peer-group relationships are an important factor in the recovery process, exposure to wide-ranging serious pathology can have an adverse effect upon recovery. Any decision to admit a patient must, therefore, come with the recognition that the admission, in and of itself, has the potential to cause harm.

The psychiatrist must make her decision in relation to her understanding of the anxiety generated in the clinical situation and in the wider dynamic situation that includes the anxiety of other professionals, the educational system, carers, and family. The adolescent patient and his disorder exist within a set of nested systems, including immediate and extended family relationships, friendship networks, school or equivalent educational provision, health services, and social services. Any decision to admit a patient to an in-patient unit is an indication that these systems are no longer able to contain the anxiety that has been generated around the patient and the disorder.

The concept of containing anxiety is again one that most psychiatrists will be aware of. As a psychoanalytic concept, it was first described by Bion (1962), referring to a function of the mother, who, in helping the infant to digest its profound anxieties, digests these anxieties herself. For example, the baby is discomfited (maybe by hunger or aloneness), and fears that he is dying. He projects these fears into the mother, who experiences them as her own: she also fears the baby is dying. She contains her fear through reverie and through seeking help from her own thought processes, the father of the baby, and so on. Having done this, she is then able to soothe the baby.

In this description, the human infant projects his anxieties into the mother, who must generally be able to both bear this onslaught and metabolise it. This metabolism or digestion of disturbing projections enables a containing transaction to pass back from mother to baby. Over time, the infant learns to bear his own anxieties through the process of having them borne by others, who, despite receiving these frightening communications, remain intact. The infant can then move towards a position of being able to contain himself, rather than having to rely on others to hold his unbearable projections. This movement from being held towards becoming able to hold oneself is a key development in establishing the infant's sense of himself as an inherently lovable being, one whose hatreds can be borne by a mother, and can, therefore, be held safely by himself, not destructively projected outwards.

Children who have not had this experience of a safe and containing mind, holding them through their development, can grow up with the sense of themselves as dangerous, unbearable, and unlovable. Children who have been taken into care will very often have had experiences of unpredictable and frightening carers, who were unable to hold themselves together, let alone their children. In the absence of an experience of containment, these children will continue to project their unbearable feelings into the people and systems that surround them, often with destructive effect.

In the case above, the patient had been through a number of placements, all of which had broken down. The psychiatrist observed the discrepancy between the boy's apparent calm and amiability and the heightened emotional state of the professionals involved in the case, rather as though the boy were at the still eye of the storm. He suggested that the boy was unable to manage his own fears and could only find relief by unconsciously putting them into those around him. Rather than agree to a therapeutic intervention, therefore, he suggested that the stability of the placement needed to be strengthened. He arranged for consultation to the care home, in order to help staff understand their feelings in relation to the young person.

The agencies involved set up a regular strategy meeting, to include reviewing risk and crisis management plans. They were able to come together to provide a model of "good enough" parenting (Winnicott, 1953) within the associated systems, and, thus, helped to fulfil the young person's need for containment. Over time, he was able to develop some skills of self-regulation. The placement held and his emergency presentations in suicidal crisis reduced altogether.

Get better or get gone

A man with a severe form of bipolar disorder was admitted to a secure unit. His condition resulted in periods lasting several weeks, during which he would be abusive, hostile, and aggressive. In between these periods, however, he was completely different. He was warm, friendly, and approachable. When well, he would have little to no memory of his "other side".

His doctor saw him at both extremes. He grew increasingly fond of the patient, as did the rest of the clinical team. Various medications could not prevent the man from becoming unwell. The doctor increasingly developed a deep sense of hopelessness. He became determined to cure the man of his dark side and introduced a new medication. This new medication was reserved for only the most severe cases and in this man's case was associated with significant risks.

The patient was not keen to take the medication but eventually, under pressure from the doctor, he did agree. The patient then deteriorated and began to refuse all medication. He became worse than he had ever been before. The doctor became consumed with a deep sense of guilt and worried that he had unknowingly harmed the patient and his relationship with him.

The area of forensic psychiatry specialises in the care and treatment of patients with mental disorders associated with significant risks to the public. The first "secure unit" designed to provide such care was Broadmoor Hospital, which was opened in 1863. Since then, the "secure estate" has expanded to include numerous units throughout the country organised into three levels of security (high, medium, and low) depending on the risks presented by the patient.

Patients enter these units either following convictions for serious crimes or due to their being considered too dangerous for "mainstream" psychiatric units. Patients in secure units generally have complex mental disorders that have not responded to conventional treatments. Such patients typically remain in the units for several years, because of the complexity of their needs and, in some cases, because of a lack of effective treatments.

These units effectively become the patient's home for a period of time, and the other patients and the professionals around them their main social network. They are often displaced significantly from their friends and relatives, and the presence of large fences erected around the units adds to a sense of being cut off from the outside world. The relationships that are formed in such an environment can give rise to strong feelings among patients and professionals alike. As a result of this, forensic psychiatry is somewhat unique. It lends itself to the forming of deep relationships between patients and professionals, often accompanied by deep and profound feelings within the professionals.

In our experience, there can be a perception among professionals that the patients who arrive into, and are contained within, the secure setting fall broadly into two types. There are those who present as unwell, receive treatment, improve, and are then discharged. These tend to be popular patients, as they cause psychiatrists, and their teams, to feel successful and potent. Conversely, there are those who are perceived as "incurable". This group of patients tend to generate feelings of hopelessness. When failure to help is associated with regular occasions of violence to others and of self-harm, feelings of hopelessness can become amplified and a sense of despair can engulf an entire clinical team. This panic and desperation can increase the tendency of the team to act in a potent way, in an attempt to counter the shared sense of futility. In such a situation, the ability of the thinking function of the team can become clouded and can fold under a pressure to "do".

The scenario described above illustrates one such example. In this case, the psychiatrist was driven to introduce a new medication against the wishes of the patient. The treatment was directed in two directions, both towards the patient and towards the psychiatrist's own intolerable feelings.

The organisation of care within secure settings is typically hierarchical, with the psychiatrist being considered to be at the top of a pyramid of clinical staff. This is reinforced by the title contained within statute of "Responsible Clinician". As is often the case when a group finds itself in difficulties, there is a tendency to try and evacuate these feelings into an authority figure, in a process reminiscent of the dynamic between children and carers. This process adds to the psychiatrist's drive to act. In addition, psychiatrists are possessed of the power to prescribe powerful medications, which have the potential to cause significant harm to a patient: this reality cannot be understated. In our experience, patients who enter secure settings are often prescribed a large number of medications, which, in many cases, can be discontinued without any notable and associated deterioration observed in the patient. In our opinion, it is of interest to consider whether there might be a correlation between the quantity of medications a patient is prescribed and the degree of hopelessness that has been experienced by other professionals before the patient was admitted.

Another response observed towards such patients is denial. Patients who are liked, but who are considered by the team to be "unfixable", can often fall out of mind. For example, a permanent member of the nursing team cannot recall any personal details of a long-stay patient, whom she has nursed for years. It is suggested that, rather than reflecting neglect or lack of interest, this can represent an unconscious attempt to deal with hopelessness by turning away.

Thus far, the discussion has described the response to patients that are generally "liked" by the clinical team. An interesting and different phenomenon is observed when the patient is disliked. A significant proportion of patients in secure settings have been deprived of prosocial role models and display dissocial attitudes. Clinical staff are commonly disrespected, intimidated, bullied, and assaulted by patients who have these underlying personality traits. These patients give rise to negative feelings of anger and repulsion. In some instances, these difficulties can be overcome, but in others they persist and can, at times, lead to similar feelings of hopelessness and despair. In these cases, however, hopelessness tends to transform into blame. Such patients might begin to be labelled, pejoratively, as "attention seek-ers", "manipulative", and "psychopaths". While there might, at times, be truth in all of these criticisms, they are often stated as an expres-sion of frustration rather than as clinically useful observations. These patients might find themselves excluded by the team. Often, this involves a reformulation of their diagnosis to create an argument that they are placed in the wrong setting. At other times, the patient might be transferred to another hospital for some seemingly minor misde-meanour. The team might then reassure each other that the move was clinically indicated, and the underlying motives might go unheard. Such instances can serve to reinforce to a patient that professionals are not to be trusted and to deepen a profound experience of rejection.

So it is that patients who engender feelings of hopelessness in the professionals around them might find themselves being passed through the system. With each move, their condition is worsened, and they might never find containment.

The current training of psychiatrists in the UK provides a good grounding for understanding medical issues, such as how medica-tions should be prescribed, how illness should be described, and how risk should be formulated. What is often lacking is an appreciation and awareness of how the feelings generated by patients affect the behaviour of the teams charged with caring for them.

Fear in the workplace

A hospital psychiatrist is contacted by a nurse, who warns him that a male patient has made a number of threats towards him. The patient has told the nurse that he has been thinking about hurting the psychiatrist for some time and, every time the psychiatrist comes on to the ward, feels close to acting on this thought. The psychiatrist is fearful and begins to find reasons to avoid the ward, resulting in other patients not getting the care they need.

The psychiatrist comes to the ward one Monday morning and discov-ers that this patient has been granted leave in the community and has assaulted a member of the public. An investigation follows and finds that the patient had been showing signs of agitation prior to the leave and should never have been allowed out.

Following the incident in the community, the patient is returned to the ward and placed in a seclusion room for a prolonged period of time.

A nurse begins to feel uneasy about this but when she raises her concerns she is met with harsh criticism from a number of staff.

Strong emotions are commonly felt in secure settings, and fear is no exception. Interestingly, although common, it is rarely discussed. Patients who enter secure settings have generally committed acts of considerable harm, such as violence, murder, and rape. The people who work alongside such patients are placed in highly vulnerable positions on a daily basis and have to experience significant levels of fear. Although a patient's access to the community is tightly controlled, they are usually afforded a considerable amount of freedom to move around within the hospital.

Aggression is a very powerful tool in society and can be an effective means of getting needs met. The term "instrumental aggression" is reserved for instances of aggression designed to intimidate and induce fear. This method is effective in hospital settings as well as in the community. Many patients lack skills in negotiation and, for them, aggression is their default approach to securing needs. Many will have witnessed this method by parents and other role models and a central challenge for the care team, once the patient has been admitted, is helping them unlearn violent methods of resolving difficulties and develop more prosocial approaches.

The responses to fear are varied and interesting to observe, as the scenario given above illustrates. The response to fear in secure settings should not be assumed to be a conscious process. Instead, it can appear that action might be taken in order to avoid awareness of any feelings at all.

One possible response to fear is avoidance. Certain professionals, like psychiatrists, who are not involved with day-to-day care, might find this easier than others. A psychiatrist who avoids his patients is likely to start neglecting core aspects of his role, resulting in poor standards of care.

However, most professionals are unable to avoid patients who elicit fear within them. This is particularly true for nurses and healthcare professionals, who spend the majority of their shift in close contact with patients. Being unable to avoid a frightening patient at work might lead a staff member to give up his job, to move on, or to become ill and take sickness leave.

Some professionals, who have to work in close proximity to frightening patients, might respond in other ways. For example, they might be cowed by their fear. In an environment that is not conducive to discussing difficult emotions, frightened professionals might find themselves playing down their fear by assessing a patient's risk to be lower than it is. If this is not challenged, the decision-making capacity of the clinical team (and the hospital) could be affected. This has the potential to lead to very dangerous situations. For example, an unsafe patient could be granted leave into the community without adequate safeguarding measures being taken. Then, when incidents do occur, subsequent analyses often indicate that a team's decision-making capacity had become compromised some time prior to the incident.

Professionals who are minimising risk might believe themselves to be acting as the patient's "advocate". They might try to persuade those around them of their own viewpoint. The drive to collude might be very strong for all concerned, including the patient, and staff who attempt to challenge a shared misapprehension of risk might find themselves cast out of the group or come under attack from colluding staff. In such a situation, the threat is felt to be to these professionals' idea of themselves as strong, competent, and caring.

Fear has the potential to become overwhelming in secure settings, which might explain why it is so rarely acknowledged. A submissive response seeks to reduce fear by avoiding conflict. Another response to feeling frightened is to defend through reciprocal aggression.

Secure settings have a number of tools at their disposal, which can be used to keep people safe. These include restraint procedures, forcible administration of medication, and seclusion areas. When used appropriately, these methods are an essential component of secure care and are intended to prevent harm to patients and staff. However, they have the potential to be used as instruments of punishment. Thus, one approach to managing fear can be to reverse the troubling situation by swapping roles, with the aim of exchanging the roles of aggressor and victim. This generally manifests through excessive medication of the aggressive patient, and prolonged and unnecessary time spent isolated in seclusion areas. This striving for position of "top dog" can enter abusive territory, a process further reinforced by an underlying belief that the patient is in some way deserving of the abuse, due to the harm she has previously inflicted on others. In some cases, this appears to be sought out by the patient, who also believes she should be punished and derives a perverse satisfaction from the experience.

As outlined above, the responses to fear are complex and varied. Fear cannot be addressed unless professionals can both recognise when they are frightened and, as importantly, be able to talk about it honestly within their teams. It is essential that staff teams should be provided with a space in which to come together and discuss the difficult feelings they might be experiencing. However, although such groups can be of immense benefit, attempts to establish them can be met with stiff resistance, as professionals might find their own vulnerabilities more frightening than the risks associated with overlooking them. So, while in secure settings, the special term known as "relational security" is reserved for issues of risk pertaining to relationships between individuals, it is by no means always the case that this recognition of the problem results in the institution of appropriate measures to manage it. Putting theory into practice remains a challenge.

Discussion

In this chapter, we have offered four examples of clinical situations, which are understood with reference to psychoanalytic ideas. The main psychoanalytic ideas referred to are transference, countertransference, and containment.

These ideas are not fully integrated into everyday psychiatric practice, although all psychiatrists, whatever their level of training or expertise, are likely to be able to give a working definition of the first two terms, and would also be likely to recognise the idea of "containing anxiety" as a key aspect of the work within the multi-disciplinary team.

While it is our opinion that these ideas cannot be understood in isolation from their original context of psychoanalytic theories of the unconscious, we do believe that both transference and countertransference, as well as the notion that anxiety can be contained by a mind capable of receiving projected anxiety, can be employed without a detailed understanding of psychoanalytic thinking. The evidence lies in the fact that they are found to be so clinically useful by psychiatrists like us, who might be psychoanalytically minded but who have not had an in-depth psychoanalytic training. Psychiatrists who might be more ambivalent about the unconscious mind could find their practice enriched by a deeper and wider understanding of the relevance of psychoanalytic concepts to clinical practice and especially for challenging relationships.

Psychoanalytic theory is non-reductive: the human mind is represented as extraordinarily complex and fundamentally unknowable. In fact, it could be said that psychoanalysis is founded on the premise that the nature of individual human beings is to be unknown, both to that individual and to those around him. This recognition of the limitations of knowing might be at odds with other models of mind and mental functioning used within psychiatry, including the predominant biomedical model. Psychoanalytic theory allows for, and expects, irrationality and unpredictability in human beings in ways that other models are often unable to do. This can be helpful in gathering an understanding of why interventions fail or do not go as expected. It can also aid clinicians in understanding their own complicated emotional reactions to their patients.

Within the framework of psychoanalysis, all of us can be considered to share in the mental pain and disturbance of our patients to a greater or lesser degree. Psychiatrists have minds, in the same way as everyone else, and they, too, are affected by their early developmental experiences. When they encounter their patients, they do so at both a conscious and an unconscious level. They might find their patients attractive or repellent, seductive or frightening. They might find themselves wishing to protect their patients or to punish them. Importantly, many of these feelings are likely to be experienced unconsciously. Therefore, the problem of the countertransference is that it is unknown and may be revealed only in what is done, rather than what is felt. It might be that understanding whether something has been enacted—which may be something good or something ill—can be found only in retrospect. Therefore, while the psychiatrist may not be fully aware of his feelings, his actions will be affected and shaped by them.

In this chapter, we have given examples of how unrecognised unconscious disturbance has the potential to give rise to harmful courses of action. We have also given examples of how whole groups of clinicians can be affected by unconscious processes and how patients might suffer if these processes are not recognised.

There are a variety of interventions available to clinicians to help them towards an understanding of how they may be affected by their patients. For example, attendance at Balint groups is a Royal College of Psychiatrists mandatory aspect of the core training for all UK psychiatrists. While there is currently no requirement for specialty trainees (higher level psychiatric trainees) or for consultants to attend such groups, this is likely to be in place in the coming years, with the increasing recognition of the developmental value of Balint groups at senior levels and as consultants increasingly seek out Balint groups. (See, for example, *Learning from the Cradle to the Grave*—a therapeutic education strategy for developing psychotherapeutic psychiatry (Johnston, 2017).)

We think that, far from being in some way immune to unconscious processes, senior psychiatrists, who occupy positions of significantly increased responsibility and increased work pressure, are as vulnerable as their trainees, or even more so. Their increased vulnerability is linked with their potential to unconsciously cause iatrogenic harm to their patients, which increases respective to their power and responsibility. We would recommend that all mental health teams, including their psychiatrists, have access to regular reflective practice groups. Reflective practice groups, if sufficiently well contained and well led, should allow honest discussion of troubling and disturbing feelings concerning patients, teams, and the systems they work in.

Difficult patients are difficult because they arouse difficult feelings. Professionals working with patients who are disturbed will experience disturbing feelings in relation to them, whether they access appropriate supervision or not. Professionals who do not have a space in which to think about this, and a theoretical model that encompasses such disturbance, might find themselves acting out their disturbance, potentially dangerously, rather than being able to recognise and work through it. It is, therefore, of crucial importance that adequate time and space are given to considering feelings generated among the team. Creating safe spaces where people can be open about feelings can go a long way towards naming some of these feelings, and preventing them from being acted out, with potential harm for patients. Reflective psychiatrists play an important role in this.

We have frequently had the experience of being approached by panicked and exhausted staff. What follows is typically a very brief description of the patient, followed quickly by the question, "What are you going to do?" In such situations, the best response may be: "Before I do, I shall listen, and then we shall think."

CHAPTER SEVEN

Working with dilemmas and disappointment in difficult places: towards a psychosocial model for team-focused reflective practice

Christopher Scanlon

> He who fights with Monsters should be careful lest
> thereby he become a monster . . .
> And if thou gaze long into the abyss, the abyss will
> gaze into thee . . .
>
> (Nietzsche, 1886, p. 146)

Introduction

I n this chapter the intention is to consider the work of those of us who choose—or for other, unconscious reasons "find ourselves" doing so—to work with traumatised people who, as a result of experiences of their early childhood neglect, deprivation, or abuse, have difficulty regulating their emotions and have a reduced capacity to mentalize (Fonagy & Bateman, 2006). However, rather than be seen as traumatised by their disadvantage and mistreatment, these service users are often experienced as difficult, unpopular, and undeserving; they attract little sympathy from the general public and so often find themselves taking up their membership of our groups and communities in ways that are problematic for themselves and/or for others

(Adlam & Scanlon, 2011; Cooper & Lousada, 2005; Gilligan, 1996; Wilkinson & Pickett, 2009).

Some of these fellow citizens seek to dominate, occupy, and subjugate others by taking up what might be called narcissistic or antisocial positions. Others take up their membership of the social in self-damaging, dangerous, and precarious ways at the edge of the group, in what we might call a borderline position. Some have attracted a formal diagnosis of "personality disorder", others might be described in terms of "complex multiple exclusion", others still might be understood (or not) more simplistically as being "the delinquent", "the deviant", "the self-harming", "the homeless", "the dangerous", and/or "the addicted". Such people will be encountered in every part of the health, education, child protection, social care, or community justice system and, as a consequence of their problematic ways of relating and behaving, they tend to become concentrated in "specialist" services and organisations that then become "difficult places" to work in.

This work, in organisations that contain high levels and concentrations of trauma and disturbance, is, therefore, characterised by uncomfortably close encounters with terrible madness, unbearable sadness, and troubling forms of badness that are, at best, too close for comfort and, at worst, reciprocally frightening. The dynamics in play are not only distressing and potentially traumatising for the individual workers, but are also corrosive of the structures and the cultures of the organisation itself. It is beyond the scope of this chapter to revisit the too numerous examples of how such traumatised organisations have become institutionally abusive of vulnerable people, or to discuss in-depth the damaging experiences of staff who are daily the subject of violence, disrespect, and abuse from their clients within these systems of care; suffice to say that neither are rare occurrences, and that, given the traumatising nature of the work, there is an ever-present risk of them happening again (and again and again) (Adlam et al., 2012; Hopper, 2003, 2011; Scanlon & Adlam, 2011a,b).

In the context of this discussion, one major and inescapable problem inherent in the work is that to look beyond the surface of patients' behavioural problems is to be immediately brought face to face with the psychosocial realities of poverty, prejudice, hatred, social exclusion, child abuse, and domestic and social violence, and to do this is always distressing and painful. On the other hand, to look away from these underlying problems and only to see the "behaviours" is to ignore the patients' essential humanity and so run the opposite risk of becoming retaliatory, neglectful, ineffective, and abusive, and this, too, is distressing and painful.

In such environments there is nowhere to run and nowhere to hide from painful encounters, and so a central aspect of the primary task of such work is to "gaze into the abyss", and to encounter this psychosocially constructed "monstrousness" without becoming "monsters". The focus of this chapter, therefore, will be on supporting staff to work with the frustrations and challenges that inevitably arise from working with difficult people in difficult places, in the hope of reducing the risk of further damage to themselves and to their patients.

Practising disappointment

If you can keep your head when all about you
Are losing theirs and blaming it on you . . .
Or being hated, don't give way to hating . . .
(Excerpts from *If*, Kipling, 1940, p. 6)

In a body of work undertaken with my colleague John Adlam (Adlam & Scanlon, 2011; Scanlon & Adlam, 2008, 2011c), we drew upon the life and times of the ancient homeless philosopher Diogenes the Cynic (Cutler, 2005; Navia, 2005) and his trenchant commentary about the inequality and unfairness that he perceived in the world surrounding him. We described how, on one occasion, Diogenes was seen begging from a statue of a goddess in the Agora and, when asked what he was doing, famously replied that he was "practising disappointment", which, we noted, is a very useful skill, both for our traumatised and traumatising patients as well as for the professional helpers who would seek to engage them.

In discussing the problem of "disappointment" from a contemporary moral philosophy perspective, Honig (1996) suggests that much professional practice takes place in what she called "dilemmatic space". Dilemmatic spaces she describes as opening up when conversations about things that do not fit together, or that contain inherent contradictions, *must* take place, and when actions are demanded that will inevitably disappoint someone. In considering this dilemmatic problem from a psychosocial perspective, Craib (1994) similarly suggests that, for many "psychosocial practitioners", having to relate to their disappointment is not a choice, and neither is it about (re)solution of problems, patient-centredness, or simple notions of "recovery". Rather, such disappointing–disappointed dynamics necessitate a capacity to work with the distressing contradictions, doubts, and uncertainties that emerge when solutions are not present and recovery is not (yet) possible. For Bion (1967), this requires that practitioners are able to contain the anxiety born of "not knowing", and to work together to develop the individual and collective resilience that is necessary to accommodate the painfulness of having to work with these reciprocal emotional, relational, and behavioural challenges and disappointments (Adlam et al., 2012; Armstrong, 2005; Hopper, 2003, 2011; Scanlon, 2012). To be able to manage these disappointments, therefore, necessitates building a systemic and organisational capacity to be with them, as problems that are an inherent part of working in the dilemmatic space, rather than seeking to solve them.

Agazarian (1997) suggests that the basic functional unit of study in any social system is not the individual but the sub-group; in this context, I propose that to think about and to manage these disappointments is a shared task, the responsibility for which lies not with the individual, but with the team. In other words, the best route to understanding the way in which any of us take up our individual membership of the group is to consider how we relate to others within the various and shifting sub-groups that we co-inhabit within that wider system. To make the group, rather than individuals, the focus of attention is also to pay due respect to the pervasive, (dis)organising social defences and group dynamics that are inherent in *all* work with difficult people in difficult places (Adlam et al., 2012; Aiyegbusi & Kelly, 2012; Armstrong & Rustin, 2014; Cooper & Lousada, 2005; Hopper, 2003, 2011; Menzies Lyth, 1988a[1959a]; Obholzer & Roberts, 1994; Scanlon & Adlam, 2011, 2012, among others).

To focus our attention on the group, or team, in these ways is also to acknowledge that none of us can easily accommodate the extent of these psychosocial processes of traumatisation on our own. So, if we are to stand any chance of managing our selves effectively in these dilemmatic conversations, not only do we have to look after ourselves, but, far more importantly, we also have to look after each other. Only then can we learn together the sort of "intelligent kindness" (Ballatt & Campling, 2010) that will enable us to relate to our patients' (and colleagues') suffering in respectful ways, and so help make our social institutions and organisations less sick places (Adlam et al., 2012; Aiyegbusi & Clarke, 2008; Campling et al., 2004; Gordon & Kirtchuk, 2008; Hopper, 2011). In these ways the necessary investment of time and money into staff health and welfare will be repaid through reductions in too-high levels of stress-related sickness absence and burnout, increased morale, enhanced resilience, greater efficiencies, greater job satisfaction, more effective recruitment and retention of staff, and better patient care.

Reflections on the psychosocially informed enabling environment

Tom Main, one of the early researchers into the nature of the therapeutic milieu, described its primary task as promoting "a *culture of enquiry* into personal, interpersonal and inter-system problems . . . of impulses, defences and relations as these are expressed and arranged socially" (Main, 1989b). In similar vein, Bion discusses the power and potency of effective groupwork by pointing out that the term can have two meanings:

> It can refer to the treatment of a number of individuals assembled for special [therapeutic] sessions, or it can refer to a planned endeavour to develop in a group the forces that lead to smoothly running co-operative activity [that are] likely to turn on the acquisition of knowledge and experience of the factors which make for a good group spirit. (Bion, 1961, p. 11)

Both of these early pioneers of a more psychosocially orientated therapeutic community model held that effective teamwork, rather than technical skill, was at the heart of the work. Their argument was that it is only through in-depth exploration of the ways in which organisational dynamics influence (sub-)group behaviour (and *vice versa*) that we can understand what helps and what hinders effective functioning at work. It is in this context that I propose a crucial question for us here: to what extent is the "culture" of any given organisation characterised by a "group spirit" that is rooted in, and informed by, this more collaborative understanding about the nature of professional work in dilemmatic spaces?

Finding ways to improve collaborative and integrated working between services and practitioners has for some time been a key aspiration of the UK government's strategy to tackle a wide range of health and social care problems. This is exemplified by recent work under the broader rubrics of psychologically informed environments (PIEs) and enabling environments (Department for Communities and Local Government, 2010; Johnson & Haigh, 2010, 2011). This essentially psychosocial work is also conceptually linked to the ideas underpinning communities of practice (Cornes et al., 2014; Lees & Meyer, 2011; Soubhi et al, 2010; Wenger, 1998), "managed clinical networks" (Ormrod et al., 2007), as well as the extensive literature emerging from the therapeutic community traditions, typified by Ballatt and Campling's (2010) excellent recent work on "intelligent kindness". It is beyond the scope of the chapter to rehearse the scope and dimensions of this valuable work in detail; however, what all have in common is a renewed interest in the importance of effective teamwork.

Over the years, a wide range of similar and different team-focused interventions has been proposed in mental health and social care contexts. However, despite being considered central to the development of these broadly defined "enabling environments", these interventions, though widely practised, are under-researched and so remain relatively poorly understood. The interventions have been given different names—such as sensitivity groups (e.g., Bramley, 1990; Haigh, 2000), staff support groups (e.g., Carson & Dennison, 2008; Hartley & Kennard, 2009; Kanas, 1986; Novakovic, 2002; Simpson, 2010), team development/consultation groups (e.g., Blumenthal et al., 2011; Carlyle & Evans, 2005; Rifkind, 1995; Thorndycraft & McCabe, 2008), Balint groups (Balint, 1957; Balint & Balint, 1961), interpersonal dynamics and multidisciplinary team work (Reiss & Kirtchuk, 2009), to name but a few.

Some terms, like "staff sensitivity groups", have fallen out of currency, while others—for instance, "staff support groups"—persevere. Perhaps this wish for support rather than sensitivity serves as a defence against the anxiety of recognising the profoundly disappointing dilemmas inherent in the work, or perhaps, more prosaically, it reflects a collective desire, in these austere times, for staff to be better supported in their work. Either way, the tension between "support" and a more reflective "sensitivity" raises important professional and ethical questions about the relationship between the work task, the staff team, the would-be staff team consultant, and the wider systems of governance.

Against this background, I propose to undertake a discussion of the nature of professional knowledge and how it is learnt and developed in the dilemmatic space. The discussion will be framed by a critical review of Schön's (1971, 1983, 1987) highly influential work on educating the reflective practitioner, and of the ways in which I have integrated this work with my own understanding of the role that I am describing as "reflective practice team development" (RPTD) consultancy.

Reflective practice and the nature of professional knowledge

In discussing the nature of skilful practice, I have elsewhere made use of Ryle's (1949) distinction between two domains of knowledge, which he described as "knowing that" and "knowing how" (Scanlon, 2002, 2012; Scanlon & Weir, 1997). Ryle described "knowing that" as having more to do with "theoretical understanding", whereas "know-how" involved what Gabbard and Wilkinson (1994) described as the capacity "to think one's own thoughts". Schön (1983) coined the term "knowing-in-action" to refer to such "know-how"; he suggested that the predominant academic and managerial paradigm, which he called the "technical–rational" approach, takes little account of these ways of knowing. Rather, for Schön, the technical–rational approach was characterised by the application of a pre-determined body of technical knowledge, embodied in sets of rational policies and procedures, within which non-rational, or unconscious, processes are not considered relevant or important and so are made invisible. Viewed through a psychosocial lens, this systemic over-reliance on more technical–rational forms of "knowing that" could also be understood to be indications and manifestations of unconscious social defences against anxiety (Armstrong & Rustin, 2015; Menzies Lyth, 1989; Obholzer & Roberts, 1994).

For example, when a disproportionate emphasis is placed on the rational and intellectual quantities of "evidence-based practice", rather than on the affective, relational, reflexive, and more qualitative "know-how" of "practice-based evidence", the effect is often to undermine clinical confidence and so to disempower and de-skill front-line practitioners. In systemic terms, Schön (1971) suggests that this is the case because, in privileging these forms of knowledge, the organisational powers-that-be imagine what happens at the front line to be ancillary, subsidiary, and peripheral to their more centralised evidential and/or managerial concerns. This is particularly problematic in the types of environment that we are discussing here because this quasirational over-reliance on defensive "technical" solutions serves to deny the essentially dilemmatic nature of the work, minimise the emotional impact of working with high concentrations of trauma and chaos, and so leave individual practitioners, and their patients, feeling helpless, isolated, vulnerable, and misunderstood (Aiyegbusi & Clarke, 2008; Aiyegbusi & Kelly, 2012; Campling et al., 2004; Gordon & Kirtchuk, 2008; Hopper, 2003, 2011).

For Schön (1971), this attempt to re-balance the power relationship between those who imagine themselves to be at the centre of these evidential and managerial discourses and those who are subject to them is not to supplant official bodies, or to deny the importance of strategic direction. Rather, the aim of empowering the front-line clinicians is so that they can work with those at "the centre" to accomplish what neither can do alone. This, of course, also means that the centralised privileging of technical–rational forms of evidence needs to be reviewed, and additional resources provided to support the front-line, so that these conditions of uncertainty and disappointment in the dilemmatic spaces can be managed more effectively. The implication is that the learning organisation (Argyris & Schön, 1974, 1978: Schön, 1971; Senge, 1990; Stacey, 2003) can only be created if "managing the business" and "learning how to learn from experience" (and from each other), though recognised as systemically related, are also viewed as distinct activities, utilising irreducible forms of knowing that need to be developed through different types of conversation in different spaces and places.

Schön (1983, 1987) suggests that this "learning from experience" has two distinct aspects: "reflection-in-action", and a lower-order set of skills that he calls "reflection-on-action". Reflection-on-action, through which practitioners learn skills from recalling past actions and/or preparing for future action, has an essentially "there-and-then" focus and typically involves the building of a more conscious, shared team narrative of the work. Reflection-*in*-action, discussed in more detail below, is when the focus is on the ways in which non-rational projective and introjective processes, which are often distressing, come to be unconsciously "held and contained" (James, 1994) within the here-and-now lived experience of the team members.

To build this reflective capacity within a team, it is vital that *all* members of the multi-disciplinary team regularly meet together. This is because patients disclose different aspects of their narratives, and project different aspects of their fragmented and split identities, into different members of the team—*all of which* it is important and necessary to understand in order to formulate a more integrated picture of their narratives and histories. For instance, some patients—perhaps those with a more grandiose sense of entitlement—might be more (un)consciously preoccupied with senior staff, while the person with a history of deprivation and neglect might be overlooked, or might identify more readily with the more junior, ancillary staff (Music, 2009). It is particularly important to enable more junior members, or ancillary staff, to speak, because they are closest to the patients, often have the most intense relationships, and so frequently have the missing pieces of the puzzle that are not available to those who are, or are experienced to be, most distant and/or least available to the patients. Clearly, extra sensitivity might be demanded of the RPTD consultant in order to encourage junior members and ancillary staff to speak, as they are often doing so against a gradient of power that makes it difficult.

While there is no doubt that encouraging active participation in "reflection-*on*-action" is necessary for the building of this shared narrative and for co-operative problem-solving, it is suggested that for team development this approach does not sufficiently take into account the ways in which the systemic social defence mechanisms, sub-grouping, and unconscious personal and group dynamics are played out. To be able to reflect-*in*-action effectively requires a different approach to the task, one that seeks to make sense of the more unconscious group and systemic dynamics and the ways in which they are transferred from the clinical context into the "here-and-now" of the team reflective space. It is to a more detailed description of this process that I now turn.

Reflection-in-action: systems,
sub-systems, and the parallel process

In any system of interrelating there is an isomorphic resonance within and across the different levels and sub-groups of this system (Agazarian, 1997; Stacey, 2003). Within complex systems of care, these different levels are represented and displayed as interactions between the managerial, staff team, and patient sub-groups, as well as in relation to the demands placed upon them by the wider social systems (including mediated public opinion). These sub-groups are, in one way or another, defined by issues of power and influence, rivalry and allegiance, dominance and submission, and other group-relational dynamics. The membership of some of these sub-groups is formally defined, for example, in terms of occupational and social grouping such as professional discipline, seniority, gender, age, ethnicity, sexuality, etc.; the membership of other sub-groups is more tacit and informal, and is revealed in relation to shared social and personal opinions, attitudes, likes and dislikes, and the relational and behavioural patterns arising from them.

For example, typically in work with patients with complex and fragmented histories, splits readily open up between those team members who see a patient (or colleague?) only as a victim, with the consequence that the patient's capacity to face up to, and work with, his/her historical and ongoing offensiveness and culpability is avoided, and so crucial aspects of their real needs are neglected. At the same time, other team members become preoccupied by the same patient's offensiveness or culpability and, thereby, neglect their victimhood. This complex process of fragmentation is made all the more complicated by other team members (often the majority), who coincidentally behave "as if" they are disinterested bystanders, watching passively as these dramas unfold. The pay-off for them is that they temporarily avoid conflict, but, in so doing, they simultaneously neglect the patient and disappoint their colleagues by not joining in (Adlam et al., 2012; Gabbard & Wilkinson, 1994; Hopper, 2003; Karpman, 1968; Scanlon & Adlam, 2011a,b). What these seemingly antagonistic positions have in common is that each, in their different ways, unconsciously seeks to avoid the contradictory and painful reality that it is rarely a simple case of "either/or", but is more often the confusing both/and case that the offensiveness of many of these patients is rooted in prior, and current, experiences of being victimised.

The situation is further complicated by the fact that, because these roles and positions are partial, they are not real, and so are untenable and shifting. The consequence of this is that, at any given time, a staff member may find him/herself aligned with the professional, social, or personal roles and attitudes of particular colleagues (or patients), and at other times in opposition to them. At one moment, a sympathy for the plight of certain patients is mobilised; at another time, there is an alignment with a wish to judge, blame, punish, or vilify; at other times it is so hard to "think our own thoughts" (Gabbard & Wilkinson, 1994) that we are all at risk of becoming detached and ceasing to care. The point is that, without the triangulation that comes of active participation in the "reflective conversation", all of us are, at different times, susceptible to being sucked into any and all of these over-simplistic roles and relationships (Redl, 1959). In this context, Luft (1982) suggests that a central aim of "learning how to learn from each other" is to provide the opportunity for individual practitioners to give and receive feedback in order to raise awareness about their "blind spots" and to talk about their valency for this type of role suction, and so take up their membership of the team in more realistically empathic and cohesive ways (Armstrong, 2005; Bion, 1961; Hopper, 2003).

A number of psychoanalytic theorists have suggested a further aspect of these systemic resonances, referring to a clinical and educational application of what has been described as the "parallel process" (Casement, 1985; Eckstein & Wallerstein, 1958, among others). This way of making sense of how a patient's historical disturbance comes to be re-enacted in the here-and-now of the clinical and supervisory encounter has long been a central part of sense-making in the therapeutic communities tradition (Jones, 1968; Main, 1989b; Norton & Dolan, 1994; Rapoport, 1960; Shine, 2010; Whiteley, 1986, among others).

To make use of the parallel process in these therapeutic milieus is to pay attention to the ways in which patients' early split-off experiences are projected into the staff (and other patients), and then taken up countertransferentially by them as part of their "organisation-in-the-mind" (Armstrong, 2005). These unconscious dynamics are subsequently personified and played out in the here-and-now relationships in the clinical and reflective spaces within the milieu. In these ways, traumatic experience, which has its roots in other times and places, is brought into the matrix of the RPTD group and becomes part of the lived experience of the staff team—and so becomes available to the type of enquiry that is reflection-in-action.

Case discussion

For example, in one RPTD group, while members were drifting in late (as usual), three members of the group who had arrived on time were overheard quietly talking to each other about a disturbing incident involving a theft from the Unit on the previous day. When all the team were seated, the *sub voce* conversation about the theft stopped, as if it were no longer important. In drawing attention to the fact that, in my mind, the group had started at the appointed time with a quiet discussion of a theft, we were able to discuss the ways in which "the team" both wanted and did not want to talk about their feelings about the young man who had perpetrated the theft. The conversation was paralysed by split positions, because they could not decide whether the young man, a much-liked ex-patient who had, once again, become psychotic as a result of relapsing into excessive drug use, was to be treated as a "thief", who needed to be prosecuted, or a "patient", who needed help. Imagining this to be an unconscious enactment in the parallel process, I suggested that, like them perhaps, the young man both wanted and did not want to talk, and that, like them, he was bringing his disturbance across the boundary in the way he did as a means of (unconsciously) provoking a conversation about "distress". This led on to a discussion in the group, in which the team could begin to talk together about their profound disappointment (anger and sadness) at having to see this young man in such a terrible state, then could begin to imagine how disappointed he might feel, and then to discuss how they might be less punitive (anger being the dominant affect) and how they might consider ways of reaching out to him in an appropriately boundaried way.

In this example, the capacity to make use of the parallel process is determined by the extent to which the team can be enabled to reflect-in-action about the ways in which patients' disturbance is unconsciously imported into the here-and-now of the RPTD group. When it works well, this thinking together takes the form of a reciprocal exchange, through which individual staff members reflect on their reactions to the material presented, and seek to generate hypotheses about what is revealed in the conversation about patients' unconscious communication; they are then better placed to export their collective reflective learning back into the therapeutic space. In these ways, the RPTD group is both a "facilitating environment" and a "transitional space" (Winnicott, 1990), relatively free from the pressures of the real world of practice, within which the disappointments and satisfactions of working in the dilemmatic space can be amplified, condensed, and more safely explored.

Figure–ground of reflection-in-action and reflection-on-action

A central educational task for the RPTD consultant is, therefore, to optimise an enabling facilitating environment within which the conversation can move between the "figure" and "ground" of reflection-*on*-action and reflection-*in*-action. In support of this aim, the RPTD consultant might sometimes want to encourage the sort of reflection-*on*-action that would focus on the manifest content, in ways that allow the emergent narratives and the rhythms of the clinical encounters to be more closely observed. Alternatively, s/he might want to encourage a more free-floating and associative conversation that could allow the impact of the tacitly contained unconscious material played out in the here-and-now of the parallel process to emerge and be explored in the group. For teams unused to this way of working, this process can be difficult, demanding, and sometimes disturbing, requiring time, effort, tolerance, and patience if it is to be put to good use. In this context, an important timely challenge for the RPTD consultant is always to seek to work in what Vygotsky (1978) calls "the zone of proximal development". That is to say, to work with the team at the closest edge of its comfort zone, in order to ensure effective "decompression" rather than provoke too much anxiety by delving too deep, too soon.

In my experience, the actual focus of the conversation does not much matter, because the primary concern of the consultant is always to make links and bridge these different sub-systems and levels of conversation. For instance, if a team begins by talking about the patients' issues, the task of the RPTD consultant is to make links to the impact and the effect of these issues on their own functioning. Conversely, if they begin by talking about their own anxieties, the task is to help them make links to how this connects to patients' anxieties and/or to the wider dynamic challenges in the organisation-as-a-whole. As discussed above, the key challenge is to be able take up a balanced stance that is sufficiently supportive and sufficiently provocative so that the group spirit is characterised by genuine curiosity, active engagement, and a willingness to explore.

In this context, I consider it important that the RPTD consultant should adopt a more mentalizing approach (Fonagy & Bateman, 2006). That is to say, an approach that seeks to be empathic, active, engaging, explanatory, linking, and informative, rather than to be overly analytic, confrontational, or interpretative. This mentalizing attitude raises further questions about the RPTD consultant's relational style, where they are positioned, and how they inhabit their authority on what Connors (1988) discussed in terms of the "observation–participation continuum". On the one hand, if the RPTD consultant is over-identified with a role that appears to be too much of an external, "blank screen" observer, rather than an active participant who is working "alongside", this is likely to be problematic. On the other hand, if over-identified with a helping or rescuing role (Karpman, 1968), s/he may be "sucked in", become less observant, and so lose authority and credibility.

To paraphrase Foulkes's (Foulkes & Anthony, 1965) dictum that group analysis is "analysis of the group, by the group—including the conductor", I might suggest, in the spirit of the literature outlined above, that the relational task of promoting a facilitating group spirit might be considered as: "reflection-*in*-and-*on*-action of the team, by the team—including the consultant".

Balancing "clinical" and "managerial" anxieties

As Drennan and colleagues (2014) point out, a further dynamic challenge for the RPTD consultant is how to take a realistically balanced position in relation to the inevitable tensions between "managerial anxieties" and "clinical anxieties". This is important because, as Maher (2009) emphasises, in unstable, or dilemmatic, contexts such as these, the primary need is *always* for sufficient resources, and the effective management of these resources, and no amount of staff support, supervision, sensitivity, or consultation can ever be a substitute, a replacement, or an apology for its inadequacies. In this context, "management" is not a *centralised* activity that is the responsibility of the designated "managers", any more than "clinical practice" is a peripheral activity that is the domain of "clinicians". Effective management in the learning organisation is a co-operative activity that requires all stakeholders to have sufficient mutual confidence to allow each other to take up their respective professional authority in empathic, respectful, and collaborative ways (Argyris & Schön, 1974, 1978; Schön, 1971, 1983; Senge, 1990; Stacey, 2003).

To do this, of course, also requires a capacity to have honest and open conversations about limited resources, and what is "good enough" in these austere times. As Simpson (2016) and Drennan and colleages (2014) observe in their different ways, these conversations are often contested, always fraught, and represent a significant dynamic challenge for the RPTD consultant. For instance, if the RPTD consultant is experienced by "clinicians" as being over-identified with managerial anxieties, s/he might be (realistically) viewed with suspicion in the clinical context. On the other hand, if s/he is, or is seen to be, over-identified with a "clinical" anxiety, s/he might be (realistically) viewed by managers as rabble-rousing. In order to pay due respect and be properly mindful of these dynamics, I suggest that it is necessary to build reflective spaces for RPTD consultants themselves to be able to think together about how to position themselves in these essentially dilemmatic conversations.

To ensure clarity of task, it is, of course, also necessary to have a clear formal contract with the employers and to have regular separate "brokerage" meetings with the designated manager/commissioners, in order to ensure that an ethical and professional balance can be struck and so all can remain "on task". The reality of these dilemmatic tensions also raises important questions about the status of the RPTD consultants, their seniority within the system, and about the organisational level at which decisions about the strategic implementation of RPTD interventions are taken.

Case discussion

In one RPTD project that I led in a large mental health Trust in London, four senior clinicians (with shared backgrounds in housing, social work, clinical psychology, group therapy, and nursing) were recruited, to an exacting job description, to provide strategically driven RPTD input into all the wards and community teams of a large forensic mental health service. All four members of this project were recruited at Consultant (Band 8c) grade and we met regularly together to reflect upon the shared work.

In my role as project lead, I reported directly to the Chief Operating Officer, and, as such, the responsibility for the project was held at the most senior level. This was helpful, because it allowed for the establishment of a feedback loop that could make connections between the "management anxiety" within the Directorate and the "clinical anxieties" of the team members as outlined above. It was also helpful because it provided the team of RPTD consultants with the credibility, the seniority, and the open channels of communication that could allow them to inform, support, and challenge both sets of anxieties and decisions, as the ethics of the situation demanded.

As might be imagined, balancing these contrasting needs and demands was a difficult "tightrope walk" (Coltart, 1992), but a precarious balance was maintained that I do not think could have been achieved if, as is often the case, the staff team consultants were appointed either in more piecemeal ways, at a more junior level, and/or by managers who are less senior within the system as a whole.

Some practical considerations pertaining
to the role of RPTD consultant

I hope that it will be clear from the discussion and analysis above that, defined in these ways, RPTD consultancy is a complex and demanding role. Further, although the professional knowledge underpinning its development is described in the literature as "psychologically informed", in my view, the skills required to undertake this complex psychosocial role do not align with the basic training of any of the traditional defined psychological therapies or related core professions. Rather, I see the development of the skills of RPTD consultancy as requiring a further and advanced, in-depth, post-graduate clinical, educational, and managerial understanding of the dynamics of working in the dilemmatic space. Here, we might also remind ourselves that Freud (1937c) suggested that there were three impossible professions: psychotherapy, education, and governance; viewed from this perspective, we might imagine this dilemmatic role to be akin to what Roberts (1994a) described as a "self-assigned impossible task". In this sense, the RPTD consultant must be prepared to suspend judgement, tolerate high levels of personal anxiety, have an ability to learn from experience and to learn from mistakes (Casement, 2002), and crucially the capacity to manage the disappointment that is inherent in the role.

Regrettably, there are too few dedicated post-graduate professional development programmes that offer specific training for this role, and so my own mistaken and disappointing professional development has involved me in building a portfolio of learning in the field. This has been enabled through seeking relatively bespoke consultation from recognised experts, being a member of a peer group with colleagues undertaking similar work, and through undertaking a range of experiential learning programmes from a variety of institutes, conferences, and organisations.

Because the bulk of these professional development opportunities are rooted in "experiential" rather than formal "academic" learning, the learning trajectory of the would-be RPTD consultant is difficult to prescribe. However, some of the organisations with an interest include: the Institute of Group Analysis (London), the Tavistock Institute for Human Relations (TIHR), the Tavistock and Portman NHS Trust, the Tavistock Consultancy Service, the Grubb Institute of Behavioural Studies, the Systems-Centred Training and Research Institute (SCTRI), the Organisation for Promoting Understanding of Society (OPUS), International Society for the Psychoanalytic Study of Organisations (ISPSO), as well as specific group relations programmes such as those organised by the Tavistock Institute for Human Relations in London and the A. K. Rice Center for the Study of Social Systems in the USA.

To summarise some of the essential knowledge and skills required for the role outlined above I would suggest that it is necessary to have:

- a high degree of credibility as a senior practitioner (this might include a qualification as a core mental health professional but could also include advanced standing as an experiential learning facilitator, action-researcher, manager, or organisational development consultant), combined with the organisational seniority to inhabit their professional authority in ways that inspire confidence in the team;

- a coherent theory of mind that includes an in-depth understanding of the operation of unconscious mental defence mechanisms, security and insecurity of attachment, reflective functioning, and mentalization;
- a systems-psychodynamic and educational appreciation of the ways and means through which people do and do not "learn from experience";
- an understanding of the impact of psychosocial processes of traumatisation, their relationship to the roles of victim, perpetrator, rescuer, bystander, and how these are played out in clinical practice and in the parallel process;
- an understanding of the operation of creative/destructive forces and basic assumption dynamics in groups and organisations;
- an in-depth appreciation of difference and diversity and the discourses of power and inclusion/exclusion in groups and organisations, for example, the difficulty of promoting participation, empowerment, and recovery in prejudicial, discriminatory, and stigmatising environments;
- an understanding of the necessary conditions that make for an "enabling environment" in a range of residential and community settings;
- a systems-psychodynamic, group-relations, and organisational understanding of "authority", "role", "leadership", "follower-ship", and "membership" in organisational life;
- sufficient personal development, self-awareness, and confidence to manage high levels of anxiety, to be able to "speak truth to power", and the capacity to support and challenge different capacities and vulnerabilities in others.

Concluding remarks

The aim of this chapter has been to describe the ways in which enabling environments can be optimised by helping individual practitioners, "working with difficult people in difficult places", to take up their professional role and their membership of the team in more confident and authoritative ways. My argument has been that the development of the necessary team-based "intelligent kindness" has less to do with individual staff members developing a technical competence, but is much more about a readiness to join and actively participate in reflective interpersonal and inter-professional conversations in the dilemmatic space.

I have suggested that, to do this effectively, some serious questions need to be addressed regarding the strategic implementation of team-focused interventions and the psychosocial focus in the basic education and training of mental health, social care, and community justice practitioners, as well as in relation to the need for further research and training in the field. I have attempted to map out some of the factors and variables that might optimise this development, and hope that I might have made some contribution to progressing these discussions.

CHAPTER EIGHT

On being an observing participant in a therapeutic institution: using psychoanalytic understanding in the work in an organisation

Wilhelm Skogstad

Introduction: a psychoanalytic view of organisations

O rganisations, shaped and run by human beings, are deeply influenced by powerful, yet largely unconscious, psychological processes. Anxieties, and defences against them, have an impact on the institutions and might undermine their very functioning. For mental health services, it is, therefore, not just individual patients who may benefit from psychoanalytic understanding, it is the services themselves that can gain a deeper perspective.

Working with people suffering from mental illness creates anxieties, which professionals have to find ways of dealing with. They do not just do so individually; the institution as a whole will find its particular way of responding to these anxieties and will create a particular culture. Defences are necessary in dealing with anxieties, on an individual and a social level, and might be helpful, but they might also be maladaptive and lead to serious dysfunctions. Psychic defences of individuals and organisational ways of functioning may come together to form a "social defence system" (Jaques, 1955). Organisations differ significantly in the culture they develop: they might be more containing and open to anxieties or might be more defensive and malfunctioning.

In the 1950s, the psychoanalyst Isabel Menzies Lyth studied the nursing system of a general hospital (Menzies Lyth, 1988b[1959b]) and found a seriously dysfunctional system based on social defences. Techniques aimed at helping individuals avoid the experience of anxiety, guilt, and uncertainty—she called them "defensive techniques"— often undermined the nurses' primary task of caring for their patients. For example, moving nurses repeatedly from ward to ward and breaking up tasks in patient care between different nurses prevented any emotional closeness between nurses and patients. While the resulting depersonalisation reduced anxiety, it also led to unsatisfactory care for patients and a lack of morale among nurses.

Conflicts are inherent to any kind of work and can cause anxieties and doubts. As Menzies Lyth showed, different poles of such conflicts may be lodged in different groups within an organisation, through the processes of splitting and projection. No longer experienced as internal conflicts, they can turn into tensions between groups. For example, different professional groups might take diametrically opposed positions or massive gulfs might open up between staff and patients. Once such divisions have become institutional realities, they are difficult to bridge and the polarisations may prevent appropriate solutions.

To give an example: working with suicidal and self-harming patients, as I have done for twenty years at the Cassel Hospital, involves facing severe anxieties and challenging conflicts, in oneself and in a team. Patients need to be protected from dangerous self-destructive impulses and staff from the terrible fallout of serious incidents. Yet, one also needs to help patients change their entrenched patterns of self-destructive behaviour and reduce their over-dependency on others. Complete avoidance of risk might be to the detriment of development in patients. Trying to push them out of their over-dependency prematurely, however, might lead to serious self-harm. It is challenging and anxiety provoking to remain in touch with these different aspects and to tolerate risks. Such conflicts and anxieties are, therefore, often avoided. Professionals may focus purely on the aim of minimising risk: all destructiveness is located in the patient, who may be Sectioned and put on continuous observation while fighting against this system. Such a division ignores the healthier side in patients and the hostility in professionals. This in turn may lead to a vicious cycle in a patient's self-destructive behaviour and to growing frustration and helplessness in staff.

Organisations carry a culture of their own. Culture is difficult to define, and yet an important aspect of the emotional life of an organisation. It is shaped by attitudes and beliefs, patterns of relationships and the psychosocial context. As Hinshelwood and I have suggested (Hinshelwood & Skogstad, 2000), culture is underpinned by shared, often unconscious "cultural attitudes" or "myths".[2] One chronic psychiatric ward seemed to harbour the myth that "any lively interaction will lead to outbreaks of madness" (Hinshelwood & Skogstad, 2000, p. 157). This was not a consciously expressed belief, but a shared unconscious phantasy that could be deduced from observed behaviour: while making efforts to enliven the social life and interpersonal relatedness on the ward, nurses continually defeated these very efforts.

There are often wider systemic processes that have a significant bearing on an organisation. Changes in the organisational structure and pressures on the wider organisation, for example, can have a massive impact. This is increasingly the case in the NHS, where budget cuts and repeated structural changes, together with performance targets and intensive monitoring, can create intolerable pressures and deep uncertainty.

The myth that "the more staff are monitored, the better they work" seems to pervade the culture of the NHS and undermines morale. My own case description that follows gives an example of such an impact of wider organisational processes.

Hinshelwood and I have described a method of observing institutions, derived from psychoanalytic infant observation (Hinshelwood & Skogstad, 2000). A particular service is observed once weekly for an hour over a period of time; one's observations and emotional reactions are written up after each session and then discussed in a seminar group. The role of observer, without direct participation or the need to carry out tasks or facilitate change, allows one to use one's eyes, ears, and mind to pick up the atmosphere of an institution, and the collective mind of a seminar group can help make sense of the observations. Through this process, defensive techniques, institutional pressures, and unconscious attitudes may be recognised and understood.

Building on the concept of "participant observer", developed in field research, we argued that such an experience might help one become what we have called an "observing participant". By that, we mean participating fully in one's professional role in an organisation with all its complicated dynamics, while also being sensitive and observant to the institutional processes one is immersed in. This might "help one to think about rather than act upon the pressures within the organisation" (Hinshelwood & Skogstad, 2000, p. 26).

In the following case study, written in 2009, I would like to give an impression of how, in my role as a consultant of an in-patient unit at the Cassel Hospital, I tried to participate and lead as well as observe.

On being an observing participant in a therapeutic institution: a case study*

The therapeutic institution and its underlying anxieties

The Cassel is a psychoanalytically orientated NHS hospital with a long history, going back to its founding in 1920. Under the psychoanalyst Tom Main, its director from 1946 to 1976, it developed into a therapeutic community based on psychoanalytic principles, and pioneered psychosocial nursing as an approach that fosters mutual care and self-responsibility (Hinshelwood & Skogstad, 1998; Main, 1989a; Skogstad, 2001, 2006). The Cassel now offers intensive treatment for patients with severe personality disorders and high levels of acting out, which has proved successful in long-term research (Chiesa et al., 2006).

The Cassel is a more complicated organisation than most therapeutic communities (Hinshelwood & Manning, 1979). Treatment of patients takes place on very different levels: individually in one-to-one psychotherapy, in small groups of two or three in the nursing

---

* This section is a slightly revised version of a paper, originally given in November 2009 at the University of Essex at a conference to mark the retirement and honour the contributions of Bob Hinshelwood. The paper in its original form was published in 2010 in the *British Journal of Psychotherapy*, 26(4): 451–457. Reproduced with the kind permission of Wiley-Blackwell.

work and between five and eight patients in group psychotherapy, in larger groups of up to fifteen patients with nurses and consultant, and in large group meetings of the whole community of patients in the hospital. Similarly, on the staff side, there is individual supervision and small group supervision of therapists or nurses, and of nurse and therapist together, as well as whole team meetings, various professional or management groups, and a weekly large group of the whole clinical staff. Structurally, there are individual units. In the past, these numbered three, adults, adolescents, families; more recently just two, a combined adult/adolescent unit, which I head, and the families unit. There is the whole hospital and, of course, the NHS Trust we belong to with its own dynamics.

In my work as head of an in-patient unit, I need to be aware of most, if not all of these levels. Were I to look only at a patient's relationship with their therapist, I would miss out important elements that emerge in their relationships with their primary nurse, the senior nurse, or myself; were I to look purely at their relationships with staff, I would risk ignoring their often extremely significant relationships with fellow patients; by focusing on individual patients alone, I would miss out important group dynamics among the patients; by concentrating purely on patients, I would ignore influential dynamics among staff.

Important anxieties that I think have had an impact on the functioning of the Cassel are related to death—death of the institution or death of individual patients. The death of the Cassel was a very real threat in 1990 (Kennedy, 2002) and has since repeatedly cropped up as a frightening possibility: only three years ago when ten beds had to be cut, and again two years ago when the Henderson Hospital closed. The death of individual patients is always an anxiety, as many of them are seriously suicidal at times. At the time of which I am writing, I had worked at the Cassel for sixteen years; there had been three suicides (one only two years previously), and many serious suicide attempts. We often work with these anxieties reflectively, but at times they become overwhelming and undermine staff's capacity to think; at other times they are ignored at our peril. These two sets of anxieties are also connected, with the danger of suicide throwing up fears that this could lead on to a downhill path, with the closure of the hospital at its end.

From stability to disturbance

Our patients, with histories of trauma, abuse, and neglect, and symptoms of self-harm and suicidality, present severe disturbance, which must be managed, individually and in the whole group. Some patients find it too difficult and leave early and there can be waves of drop-outs. For some time, until recently, we had a stable situation, a whole year of a full unit with no drop-outs. In my own mind, I had linked this stability with my good working relationship with the unit's senior nurse, Sandra. Patients seemed to experience us mostly as a caring, firm parental couple. This was touchingly demonstrated at Christmas, when they performed, as part of our traditional event, a version of "The Twelve Days of Christmas"; the verses ended with "two wake-up calls" from Sandra and the refrain "Sir Skogstad is going to meet you".

It was, therefore, a great blow to patients, staff, and to me personally when Sandra announced she would leave the hospital. While we were very aware, as a staff team, of the great loss, we felt confident that we were strong enough to go on working as well and stably as we had done. The patients, too, seemed in touch with this loss and gave her a warm farewell, without becoming overly disturbed.

However, something very different started the following week. There was a sudden increase in patients' disturbance and destructive behaviour that took me by surprise. Some young people self-harmed repeatedly in the next few weeks; on a number of occasions, adolescents went out drinking or brought alcohol into the hospital; one day a seventeen-year-old tried to strangle herself in a very dangerous way. Three adolescents had to be temporarily transferred to an acute unit: one because her voices telling her to harm children became too strong, two because they were too suicidal. One weekend, two female adolescents took drugs with a stranger and ended up having sex with him. A group of young people made fun of another teenager by placing denigrating pictures on Facebook, and, in the young persons psychotherapy group, there was often manic excitement with relentless attacks on the therapists. A gang culture had developed among the young people and was getting out of control; the adult patients complained bitterly about them.

Observing and understanding the dynamics

How could we understand this wave of acting out and gang culture? Was it just a coincidence of individual patients' problems emerging at the same time? Was it a massive group reaction to the loss of the senior nurse? Or were there wider, more complicated dynamics?

Of course, individual patients brought their particular pathology to the situation, which needed to be understood. One of the adolescents, Andrea, who engaged in drinking and self-harm, had been deeply neglected by parents who pretended to be very caring. This might have coloured her experience of the senior nurse's leaving. Another, Beatrice, who tried to strangle herself, had broken down after her grandmother's sudden death. She was very sensitive to loss and had only recently lost the safety and relationships of the adolescent unit she had stayed in for a year. A young woman, Charlotte, who was central in the ganging up, seemed identified with her father, who led the life of a gangster; internally she showed a destructive narcissistic gang, in Rosenfeld's (1971) sense,[3] which she now externalised. And Dora, the seventeen-year-old who heard voices telling her to harm children, had been severely abused as a child while seeing her younger brother grow up unharmed. She had tolerated her voices for a while but could no longer do so when a boy from the families unit became highly intrusive, making her feel unprotected from her envy and sadism.

Yet, the individuals' pathology did not seem sufficient to explain the disturbance. Apart from Sandra's leaving, other things were happening for patients. Within a few weeks, four adult patients had reached the end of their treatment and three adolescents were admitted. This shifted the balance suddenly to a majority of adolescents, many of whom were in their vulnerable initial period. It was as if patients were, at the same time, abandoned by a parent and faced with new siblings craving for attention. Only two weeks after Sandra's leaving, my senior psychotherapist announced that she would be away for a period of time, which affected individual patients and a psychotherapy group; this caused upset and increased their sense of abandonment. I hoped the arrival of the new senior nurse, Helen, would change the situation, and yet, with her initial, rather confrontational approach, she was not experienced as the longed-for mother but more like father's new wife who attempted to reign over the house. There were also events in the wider hospital. Within a few weeks, the courts decided that the children of three mothers on the families unit should be removed and put up for adoption, in one case against the unit's recommendation. Children were very much part of the community and a source of identification. Separations, even if justified, were, therefore, very painful; having a few in a short time felt traumatic.

Looking at the staff, they, too, felt bereft by the loss of the senior nurse. On the first day without her, I noticed how anxious I was myself, more than I had anticipated; I was also worried about my senior psychotherapist's absence. The staff team soon seemed changed; there was bickering, impatient interrupting, and a previously unknown degree of rivalry. When Helen, the new senior nurse, started, she showed a manner that felt quite authoritarian, unlike the collegial tone we were used to, and this seemed to antagonise and unsettle staff, myself included. There were also changes on another level of the organisation: the Care Quality Commission[4] had investigated and severely criticised the Trust and this had led to the chief executive's sudden departure; his replacement was given the task of sorting the institution out. This had largely gone unnoticed, but when the new chief executive came to speak to the hospital staff, many were left with the worrying impression that we were being scrutinised and put under pressure from above.

All these experiences meant that, at different levels of the organisation, staff and patients had an experience of parents who were failing or abandoning them—a sense of being left alone, unprotected and vulnerable. The gang culture that developed among the adolescents appeared to me as a massive defence against the experience of vulnerability and the loss of a parent, which was experienced, consciously or unconsciously, not only by the adolescents, but more widely by patients and staff. At the same time, the ganging up and acting out were a cry for a caring and firm parental couple who could exert authority and stand up to the destructiveness in them that they themselves sensed was getting out of hand.

Such thoughtfulness and firmness is what I, with my team, aspired to provide, in dealing with patients on an individual and group level and with colleagues and the team. I had to handle my own strong feelings about the changes. Reflecting on Helen's somewhat authoritarian approach, I was able to realise how much she was driven by anxiety over her new role and responsibility and by a fear of being rejected as the new nurse. This helped me curb my initial impulse to be critical and instead to relate to her in a supportive and containing way. Reflective group meetings of the team helped us think about our anxieties, which underlay the tensions in the team, and about the dynamics among patients. We were gradually able to reinstate the boundaries that had been eroded and stand up to the destructive culture in meetings with patients. I felt we were beginning to get to grips with these difficult and, at times, overwhelming dynamics.

Dynamics on a higher level

Then, out of the blue, I received a letter from my manager. It was copied to others in my team, as well as to senior hospital staff and Trust managers. In his letter, he expressed grave concern about the number of incidents and asked us to carry out an investigation into the incidents and how they were handled. I felt attacked and undermined. Instead of speaking to me, let alone trying to help the team think about the dynamics, he had created a situation in which we had to justify ourselves, to him and to the Trust. A sense of persecution and anxiety developed in my team. In a meeting with him and our head of service, I felt I was being threatened. However, I also sensed a real anxiety in him. He seemed caught up in the fear of a major incident and of Trust managers on his own back. Without trying to contain his anxieties, he had passed them on, both to me and to my team. This could have been taken as an individual problem but I thought it might be a reaction to the changed condition of the Trust and the scrutiny we were all under. My initial impulse to say no to his demand did not seem an option in this situation; it would only have increased his anxiety and would, thereby, have escalated the problem, leading to an involvement of higher levels of the Trust.

I had to find a way of allaying my manager's anxiety and ensuring his request would be honoured while, at the same time, trying to prevent a situation in which my team and I would be likely to feel overly anxious and uncontained. I might not have managed that without the help of thoughtful colleagues, but in the end I produced a report, which showed my understanding of the underlying dynamics and our management of individual patients and the whole group. Presenting this report to the senior managers started a process that led to clearer support of my position and the risks I was taking.

Conclusion

I hope I have given a flavour of how I try, in my work, to be both a participant and an observer. Unlike many in the NHS, I have the privilege of working with colleagues who are experienced, thoughtful, and able to observe themselves, in an institution where such thinking has a shared value, even if it is not always practised.

Main (1989a) created the term "culture of enquiry" as a model for examining, understanding, and resolving the "tensions and defensive use of roles that are inevitable in any total system" (1989a, p. 136). This seems to envisage an institution where everyone participates as well as observes. Griffiths and Hinshelwood (2001) have described how such a culture can be defensively undermined, even in an institution that advocates thoughtful enquiry as a continuous task for itself. Main (1967) has also described how a creative thought can move, in a "hierarchical promotion", from the realm of the ego to that of the superego, from a useful idea to a religious belief that needs to be strictly adhered to. The idea of a culture of enquiry, based on a capacity to be curious and inquisitive, can itself move into the realm of a persecutory superego, and frequently does so in today's culture of targets and league tables, in which there is often a sense of "right" and "wrong", success and failure.

I experienced my manager's demand for an investigation as just such a superego and anxiety-driven enterprise, which I needed to respond to, counter to my initial reaction, by bringing it back into the realm of a thoughtful ego. I remembered Main's (1989a) description of the failure of the first Northfield experiment, where Bion, while successful on the lower-order level of the ward, ignored the higher-order level of the military hospital, and ended up being sacked. Therefore, I thought I had better observe not only the level I participate in directly, but the one above it as well.

Afterthoughts

Since I wrote this paper in 2009, there have been major changes and developments, both at the Cassel and in the NHS Trust it is part of. In 2011, the families unit of the Cassel Hospital had to close, due to pressures of public funding. A passionately fought campaign could not prevent a massive cull: only fifteen of the hospital's forty beds remained, and many staff, including the lead clinician, were made redundant. The Cassel was reduced to one in-patient unit and the out-patient service. I became clinical lead, at a point when the hospital's future was in serious doubt (Skogstad, 2012). In the meantime, the remaining small hospital has established itself again and its future appears, for now, reasonably secure (Skogstad, 2014). Of course, in the current political and economic climate, such a situation might change radically again at some point.

The closure of the families unit, only a few years after an earlier cut,[5] created deep fears of complete closure in the remaining staff. The death of the organisation, which had been an important undercurrent in the hospital's life for some time, now seemed a real risk. Even when, after a while, genuine grounds for optimism emerged, some staff seemed to see the hospital's presence and future in a very gloomy light—as if it were too dangerous to have hope. I thought a deeper reason for that lay in a sense of guilt for surviving the serious cuts and redundancies; this was, understandably, strongest in the nurses, who had always been, to some degree, working across units.

It needed hard work, managerially as well as emotionally, to turn things around. Within the hospital, it meant fostering hope and enthu-siasm in staff to shape the service in a new way, while accepting some harsh realities. In relation to the Trust, we needed to gather support from senior management and build trust in our capacity to make this work. Towards the outside, we needed to promote the service to refer-rers and commissioners, many of whom thought the whole hospital had closed. All this was only possible because there was, in me and in most staff, a deep conviction in the value of our psychoanalytically based approach.

After a while it became noticeable that the service was more contained than it had been before the part-closure. Acting out, although an inevitable part of working with such patients, was less frequent; such a massive wave of acting out, as described in this paper, did not occur again until recently, when my own departure brought new turmoil.

My explanation for this was twofold: the simpler organisational structure, with one in-patient unit, a clearer line of authority, and, hence, no conflicts between units with different demands, made it easier to contain the organisation; and the thoughtful working rela-tionship of the "managing pair" (myself as clinical lead and the service manager) provided a containing "parental couple" for the whole hospital, which facilitated a positive culture within the organisation.

Like other services in the NHS, the Cassel has had to struggle with the increasing demands of performance monitoring and quality control systems as well as the tightening screw of financial cuts. Performance targets, audits, and quality improvement measures are meant to secure quality of care and foster improvement. Yet, in my experience, they often only create the impression of doing so and might even undermine the clinical work. The "auditable surface" (Cummins, 2002) of measurable indicators can get confused with the reality of the clinical work it is meant to represent. A persecutory culture can develop that encourages "conformance rather than performance" (Hoggett, 2010, p. 60). Paradoxically, such a system may show "improvements", even when the reality is deteriorating (Hoggett, 2010).

A striking example of this social defence was the Trust's response to the announcement of another visit by the Care Quality Commission (CQC). For half a year, leading up to the visit, the Trust's main focus seemed to be on creating an *image* of good clinical work and preparing staff to convey this image to the CQC. Attending to this virtual reality took so much time and effort and drew the focus so much away from the task of looking after patients that it even undermined clinical and managerial work.

In this "perverse social structure" (Hoggett, 2010), financial cuts, which often lead to the loss of vital staff and containing structures, are called "cost improvement programmes"(CIPs). This is not just a euphemism; I think it reflects an omnipotent phantasy, the "myth", that one can constantly provide more for less, that services can be continuously improved while the money spent on them is going down.

I see this as a social defence system, in which anxiety and guilt are pushed downwards in the hierarchy. Instead of politicians and top managers taking responsibility and tolerating guilt for the damage created by the severe cuts they impose, problems tend to be blamed on failing managers, inadequate nurses, etc. This is the very opposite of a containing culture: anxiety and guilt, instead of being contained by senior staff, are pushed downwards, creating a deep burden and sense of persecution in middle managers and front-line clinical staff, and undermining clinical care.

It is very hard in such a system to maintain a thoughtful practice, to focus on the quality of clinical work and on containment rather than the demands of a virtual reality. As described in my paper, one needs to attend not only to the anxiety of the staff one leads but very much also to the anxiety of managers further up in the hierarchy. Refusing to participate in this system would increase their anxiety, and the pressure coming from above. Identifying with the system, however, might make one lose touch with the complex realities of one's clinical work. The only solution I see is working with the system to some degree while maintaining a "third position" (Britton, 1989).

According to Britton, a third position comes into existence when a child can recognise the link between its parents, and observe their relationship. This "provides us with a capacity for seeing ourselves in interaction with others and for entertaining another point of view whilst retaining our own, for reflecting on ourselves whilst being ourselves" (p. 87). From this position, one can recognise, and empathise with, the anxieties involved, without being drawn in by the system. This might require challenging the false assumptions involved, standing up to some of the unhelpful demands, and pointing out where they are undermining, even destructive. In this way, one might protect the culture of one's institution and the quality of one's clinical work at least from some, though not all, of these pressures.

CHAPTER NINE

A view from a death: understanding the impact on staff of mental health work with older adults

Alison Vaspe

Introduction

This chapter draws on the work of an in-house psychotherapy service for mental health staff in order to consider the case of a senior staff nurse working with older adults, who was called upon to witness a death, and who was then the subject of an enquiry regarding her failure to attempt resuscitation. From this, there is an exploration of the psychological needs and potential vulnerability of mental health staff, whose motivation for entering into the work of care often relates to their own personal experiences. It is suggested that the need to care can have a vicarious and a reparative element, with problematic consequences if staff are inadequately supported in their work, or even feel prevented from carrying out their "self-assigned impossible task" (Roberts, 1994a). The context is a post-Francis Report era, in which concerns about abuse of vulnerable patients are to the fore, but reports of failures of compassion, or worse, remain headline news.

A note on the provision of in-house psychotherapy for mental health staff

Counselling or psychotherapy services for NHS staff can be criticised for sidelining the problems of staff, rather than looking at broader, systemic problems. I suggest that therapeutic work with individuals has an important contribution to make to good workplace functioning, alongside other contributions such as thoughtful, intelligent management, reflective practice groups, clinical and managerial supervision, and organisational consultancy. All these, in different ways, constitute a resource for staff who need to use their thinking minds to work with mental health problems, in a way that is both sensitive to suffering and also robust in the face of challenging and disturbing dynamics. The value of an in-house service is that it allows a virtuous cycle to operate, moving between therapeutic work with individual staff and consultations to senior managers, informed by the work of therapy but maintaining complete privacy and confidentiality on behalf of those staff seen as therapeutic patients. A key aim of the service in question was to support staff in taking concerns back to the workplace, encouraging better relationships within teams and between staff and management.

This was an unusual service, in that the manager, herself a highly qualified psychoanalytic psychotherapist with extensive NHS experience, insisted on employing similarly qualified therapists to offer counselling to staff. Her empathy for those carrying out the difficult work of mental health, and her firmness of purpose when it came to maintaining boundaries of confidentiality and privacy, were rewarded by high organisational confidence in the service.

The service was available to the diverse range of staff employed by the organisation, including senior managers and clinicians, unqualified nurses and healthcare workers, administrative staff, security personnel, and those looking after the grounds and the buildings. This wide exposure to the workforce grounded the service in the complex life of the organisation, and, importantly, helped its therapists to maintain neutrality in situations that could evoke powerful emotions on behalf of individuals. Alongside this, the close-up of therapeutic interactions, paying attention to unconscious communication, afforded a view of the workplace that could be described as "binocular", in Bion's usage of the term:

The analyst is therefore in the position of one, who, thanks to the power of 'binocular' perception and consequent correlation that possession of a capacity for conscious and unconscious thought confers, is able to form models and abstractions that serve in elucidating the patient's inability to do the same. (Bion, 1962, p. 104)

The "patient", in this instance, could be said to be both the individual member of staff and the organisation as a whole, or parts of it.

The service operated in a very different way from the IAPT system. Rather than progressing in steps from less to more intensive therapy, highly trained therapists were the first port of call. This can be seen to make economic sense when working with staff. Prompt, in-depth attention to need that can be acute, following a personal or workplace incident, can help staff remain at work, or return more quickly from sickness absence. In addition, the therapists' level of training helped when gaining the respect of all levels of staff, including many senior and seasoned mental health clinicians, leading to consistently good service usage. The psychoanalytic form of brief, time-limited therapy employed could refer to a significant evidence base,[6] and also represented a way of thinking about experience that was familiar to many mental health staff, for example as part of their training, personal therapy, group relations events, supervision, reflective practice groups, and other forms of CPD.

For such a service to keep the trust of staff, it is essential that it should operate within a strict boundary of confidentiality. Many of those seeking help are fearful of losing the clear demarcation separating them from their patients. To be exposed as needing help with emotional or psychological distress, for instance by reports on attendance finding their way outside of the therapeutic relationship, would increase anxiety. Access needs to be direct, rather than via referral (by, for instance, occupational health or a manager). Garelick's understanding of the difficulty for doctors acknowledging their need for therapeutic help can be applied to mental health staff: for them, too, "triage" is an unhelpful model:

An essential aspect of bespoke services for doctors is the removal of barriers to engagement . . . This is quite different from the provision of services to the general population, where triage is used at the point of entry, in part to manage demand on services. Doctors who need access to services do not need triage since they generally avoid seeking help;

the problem is encouraging them to come in the first place. People tend to suffer for some years before approaching services. (Garelick, 2012, p. 82)

The service guarantee of confidentiality extended to note- and record-keeping. The guidelines provided by the British Psycho-analytic Council (BPC), which is a professional body overseeing psychoanalytic psychotherapy practice, emphasise how necessary it is that, in the course of therapy, patients can speak freely about their problems, safe in the knowledge that the information they divulge will not appear on any records.[7] While this can be disappointing for managers (and, occasionally, for staff themselves, who might wish for a report from the service, or support for legal claims based on infor-mation from their notes), in practice, any frustration or disappoint-ment relating to this commitment to complete confidentiality seemed to be outweighed by appreciation of a service that was trusted and respected.

As well as the essential need for confidentiality, the BPC raises a legal issue about the status of notes as information:

Psychoanalytic psychotherapy is based on theories about the ways in which conscious thought and behaviour is influenced by unconscious mental activity; this activity often producing symptoms and difficul-ties. The psychoanalytic psychotherapist tries to bring these uncon-scious elements into conscious awareness ... To understand the patient ... the psychoanalytic psychotherapist takes an interest in the patients' dreams and fantasies and ... will ask the patient to say what-ever comes to mind, to free associate; this encourages uncensored irra-tional thought. *Free associations, fantasies and dreams cannot be thought of as hidden versions of objective truth ... and the patient's communications and behaviour have to be understood within the context of this relationship.*

The purpose of psychoanalytic psychotherapy is to help patients recognise and take responsibility for their ways of thinking, feeling and behaving, including previously unrecognised, unacknowledged aspects of their personalities. (www.bpc.org.uk, my emphasis)

All this is relevant to the discussion that follows, which draws on the therapy of a senior mental health nurse, who felt scapegoated and traumatised during an enquiry into an incident in which she was involved. The therapist worked to restore the nurse's capacity to think about her experience, and to re-establish a constructive relationship with the enquiry process. One regret this nurse expressed was the absence of any "de-briefing" following the incident, or of a systemic attempt to understand what had led up to it. Therapy was not intended to replace this, but to support the nurse's thinking to a point where she herself could raise her concerns, in the hope that the workplace could then benefit from taking back some of its own failings.

Both Nurse A's identity and her experiences have been disguised, to preserve anonymity, but it is also important to note that the account relies on her subjective memory of certain events, and on the subjective memory of the therapist who worked with her. These events are offered, not as objective fact, but as material for reflection on some key themes for mental health workers today.

I am grateful to Nurse A for permission to tell her story.

Death of an older adult

One night, on a long-stay mental health ward for the elderly, a man died. The exact circumstances surrounding his death were not clear, but he had for some time been physically very unwell and his death, apparently, was anticipated.

Nurse A, a senior staff nurse, who did not work on the ward in question but was available to its staff, was called to the bed of this man, who, to her trained eye, had been dead for some time. A doctor had been called.

This nurse performed some tests to assure herself that there were no signs of life.

She then realised that she had not looked at the patient's notes and that they were not where she would have expected to find them.

When she eventually found the notes, she saw, to her dismay, that there was no "Do not resuscitate" (DNR) agreement, as she had expected. No such agreement had been made with the next of kin.[8]

The doctor declared the patient dead when he arrived. Neither he, nor the coroner's report, found anything untoward in the circumstances of this death. However, the family was unhappy about it and an enquiry was initiated. Nurse A was one of the staff under investigation, because she had not attempted resuscitation while waiting for the doctor to declare the patient formally dead.

For the duration of this enquiry, Nurse A was suspended from her substantive duties. Effectively, she became a health care assistant (HCA). Another nurse, who was on duty when the patient was alive, was also investigated, but went off sick before the enquiry began and then resigned from her job.

Neither at this point, nor at any other, did Nurse A feel regret that she had not attempted to resuscitate the elderly patient. What she did feel was sorrow that she had not been able to tend to the body in her normal way, because of the turn of events following the discovery that no DNR agreement had been signed.

Nurse A believed she was being made an example of, because the other nurse was no longer present to share the scrutiny of the enquiry, the focus of which was now Nurse A's failure to attempt to revive what to her trained eye was a corpse. Her managers told her she had no cause to worry, but this did not reassure Nurse A, who was very anxious.

The enquiry lasted two years, after which Nurse A was found culpable for not trying to resuscitate the patient. She was considered to have served out her suspension, apart from six weeks, when she was not allowed into work and was unpaid. Following this, she was required to undertake further training before she could be allowed to work again. She was told she had robbed an elderly man of his potential full lifespan.

The therapeutic process: working through negative, traumatic transferences

The sequence of events described above was told to Nurse A's therapist over a period of two years. (For the most part, the service offered staff six sessions of counselling. However, there was flexibility to extend this, sometimes significantly, for cases where circumstances such as an enquiry and/or clinical need were considered to warrant it. After the initial six sessions, meetings with Nurse A were not weekly, but took place every three weeks or so.) Nurse A was very distressed and, at times, physically ill, her blood pressure rising to dangerous levels. At other times, she felt afraid that she was losing her mind. There were times when she needed to take sickness leave, but mostly she was able to remain at work. The therapeutic contribution was of an analytic relationship, which, as it developed, helped Nurse A to think about her emotional experience and her situation.

Despite having referred herself to the service, Nurse A initially found it difficult to trust the therapist. In her first session, she seemed to flinch at any questions asked. In place of a positive transference, in which the therapist might have been experienced as a helpful, sympathetic presence, there was a clear negative transference, in the course of which Nurse A called her by the name of the woman who had questioned her during the initial phase of the enquiry. It was clear that this "interrogation", as Nurse A called it, was experienced as traumatic, However, the therapist knew that, if she wanted to work with Nurse A, she needed to hear more about what had happened on the night in question, and to understand Nurse A's frame of mind, both then and now.

The therapist drew attention to Nurse A's Freudian slip of calling her by the wrong name. She suggested that perhaps Nurse A was seeing her, too, in the role of an interrogator—there to judge rather than try to understand something. When Nurse A returned for her next session, she let the therapist know that she had been looking forward to coming back. Without the chance to speak, she said, she felt in danger of going mad.

The therapist had experience of working with staff under investigation, and was familiar with the intense feelings of helplessness and frustration that often accompany the process. However, she also felt there was something she did not understand about Nurse A's situation. Then, some weeks into her therapy, Nurse A spoke of an event that had occurred immediately before the patient's death, when she had been on holiday visiting family in her country of origin. During this time, an uncle died, and Nurse A was the one to find his body. She described feeling shocked and powerless to do anything for him— even to offer her nursing ritual of care by closing his eyes. She told her therapist that, when she found the patient's body on the ward, she had experienced a powerful memory, like a flashback, of finding her uncle, dead.

Now Nurse A began to share more of her own story with the therapist, telling her of her upbringing in an African country. Her nurse training gave her the means to support her family as a single mother, after she left an abusive husband. She applied for work in the UK, where she began to specialise in mental health work with the elderly, and sent money home to her adult children and their families. She had recently begun to think about her retirement.

Nurse A also told the therapist a little about her childhood. She described her relationship with her mother as good, but with times when, for no reason that she could understand, her mother would fall silent and cease all communication for long periods. Nurse A, already a studious child, seemed to find a solution to this by working even harder, trying to do even better at school. Later, after deciding to leave her husband, she found inspiration and a vocation in her training and her work experience in the UK. She was a keen mentor and educator, who held learning to be sacred.

The experience with her uncle, but also with her mother, which was difficult for Nurse A to speak about, seemed to the therapist to have a clear relevance to the situation she was living through. She suggested that Nurse A felt the hospital was turning its back on her, like her emotionally absent mother, offering empty reassurances, but not the information and support she wanted.

Following this, Nurse A brought a dream to a session, which gave expression to the psychic confusion she was experiencing in the face of her displacement from a professional role that helped her to feel empowered, useful, and, perhaps, vicariously cared for through being able to care for others.

The dream gave an insight into feelings about a mother figure, who was not just failing her on a deep emotional level, but was actively attacking her:

> In the dream, Nurse A went into her mother's bedroom. Her mother was standing there with a cat in her arms, which sprang at Nurse A. She flinched aside in time for the cat to miss her but woke feeling terrified.

Reflecting on this dream, the therapist made a link between the present situation and Nurse A's life as a child. She suggested that, while highly condensed, and terrifying to Nurse A, the dream was helpful in offering a narrative through which they could recognise the importance to her of holding on to a sense of care in her life, through her work. She also suggested that Nurse A felt anxious in relation to herself: the trust she was beginning to feel for the therapist was fragile, as for a mother who at any point might turn her back on her—or even attack her.

The therapist wondered if Nurse A's shock on finding her uncle's body confronted her with a traumatic clash of two worlds: her professional caring role, which helped to protect her from private distress, and her private emotional life, including aspects of her past which she had buried deep in her subconscious. The flashback she experienced on finding the body of another elderly man led to the loss of her sense of vocational containment within the maternal function of the hospital. This then led to the waking nightmare of the enquiry. The therapist thought that Nurse A now felt herself, horrifyingly, to be somewhere she should not have been, as though a veil had been torn, revealing that the hospital she worked in was, in unconscious representation, her mother's bedroom; as a consequence, she felt she was being subjected to an attack, in the form of the enquiry. In order to save herself, she stepped aside, using another defence, of dissociation. Thinking about her in these terms helped the therapist to understand the strange experience of being with Nurse A, in which she felt both present but also absent, trusted, but also feared.

Another level of distress for Nurse A related to feeling painfully exposed, publicly disgraced, and helpless. Instead of being in charge of nursing standards, she was dependent on an enquiry process, over which she had no control. She reported conversations with managers, which seemed to her to be offering nothing but empty reassurance, and no solid information, especially regarding timing. The saving grace was in still being able to care, and the therapist felt touched by the intimacy of this nurse's feeling for her elderly, withdrawn, confused patients. A stickler for things being done properly, she also had stories to tell of going beyond the call of duty, from small considerations, such as knowing who liked a second cup of tea in the morning, to making extraordinary efforts, as in the past, when she had arranged an excursion for a patient who longed to visit a special place from childhood, following which the consultant psychiatrist said, "I don't know what you've done to this patient, Nurse A, but she's a different person."

Furthermore, Nurse A's new role as, effectively, an HCA, distanced her from former colleagues. She described her view of them sitting the other side of the windows in their nursing stations, immersed in their "endless paperwork" on the computers, screened from the messy, intimate tasks carried out by herself and the HCAs. Though sympathetic to Nurse A, the therapist wondered at her rather judgemental tone when speaking about these former colleagues, especially as she, too, felt uncomfortably remote from her patient, as though on the wrong side of a psychological screen that prevented close contact between them. Drawing on what Nurse A had told her of her history, she suggested that Nurse A might be seeing her, too, as remote and screened off from her experiences—a white woman employed by the same establishment that was carrying out the investigation into Nurse A, a black nurse.

This shocked Nurse A, who spoke, painfully, of how much her work at this hospital had meant to her. She felt great respect for some of those who had trained her. Clearly, she modelled herself on their values and standards. She also confessed to occasional suspicions that now she was being targeted in a way that was racist. She said she felt ashamed to have these thoughts, but the therapist wondered if she was also anxious about them and felt a need to try to placate her.

Nurse A's criticisms of the nurses continued. She thought the paperwork they had to do gave them a cleaned-up version of reality, while she had always involved herself in the patients' personal feelings and experiences. One day, she began to talk about ways in which corners were being cut, on a ward where staff were struggling to carry out their daily workload. Nurse A said she herself was feeling the exhaustion of trying to meet all that was expected of her, dreading the start of each day and returning home after her shift too tired to do anything but sleep.

Among other ways in which she described the ward falling short, one in particular stood out: the elderly men and women, she said, were having to take their afternoon nap on hard dining-room chairs, because all the armchairs had been removed from the communal rooms. Her nurse's eye bore witness to the effects of hard surfaces on thin skins, the danger of pressure sores, and the lack of comfort and cushioning for old bones.

What Nurse A was describing resonated with other accounts the therapist was hearing from staff, in which the need to make savings resulted in reduced time to spend with patients, sometimes in an increase of situations that were dangerous for the staff, and sometimes in heightened stress levels, leading staff to take sickness absence, which then could reduce staffing levels and exacerbate these problems, in a vicious circle.

As the therapist was thinking, privately, along these lines, Nurse A raised the issue of "whistleblowing", as something she felt impelled to consider.

The therapist was aware that whistleblowing was, at least on the surface, politically, being encouraged. While nothing Nurse A had said suggested that patients were being actively abused, she was describing something wrong with the treatment of elderly mental health patients, who would have limited capacity to speak for themselves. She thought, privately, that Nurse A's predicament could be made worse if she took the line of whistleblowing, but she also wondered how all this related to Nurse A's own situation. Could the situation of the hard chairs represent the ongoing enquiry, which felt so painfully rigid and unyielding?

When the therapist made this link, Nurse A fell silent. Then she began to think aloud about why the armchairs might have been removed in the context of too few staff to keep them clean and free of the smell of urine, and, hence, the risk of the ward failing an inspection on grounds of hygiene. Perhaps they were due to be replaced and there was a hiatus in the process. She reflected on the damage that could result from breaching a protective layer of standards that were acceptable, at least on paper, behind which the staff on the wards were perhaps doing their best to offer a basic level of care and protection during tough times. Instead of acting in a rash way, which could have had consequences for her and for the ward, she began to engage in an internal weighing up of the organisation's efforts to get things right, and so continue to function, and the extent to which she was in danger of allowing her emotions to drive her to a form of action that could have negative consequences. Later, she told the therapist that she thought she had been feeling an angry desire to act—to short-cut the slow process of the investigation—out of "spite", as she put it.

The psychoanalyst David Morgan works with the organisation Whistleblowers UK (WBUK). He addresses (Morgan, 2014) the complex issues surrounding the decision to speak out about problems witnessed while working for society's institutions:

> Everyday Whistleblowers, those whose name does not become a public entity, experience loss, not gain, through their decision to disclose. And whatever it is that they disclose, in all the many fields these people emerge from, the whistleblowers that I have met are waiting to have, or have had, their pension rights, mortgages and jobs

rescinded, their comfortable places of esteem in their communities dismantled, and, equally importantly, from a psychological point of view, they have lost their peace of mind and quite often their own faith in their own value and motives . . .

Of course, not all whistleblowing is benign or altruistically motivated. HMRC has an anonymous phone line for people to report tax evasion and it is apparently consistently used to denounce neighbours and family members. While disclosure can be an altruistic act it can all too easily be used for revenge and humiliation. At times, some whistle-blowers are clearly eager to attack authorities through resentment. (Morgan, 2014)

Nurse A seemed freer within herself following this discussion, and began to allow her frustration with the therapist to show. One frustration was that the therapist was not a nurse, which became a sign of difference between them: as with the enquiry process, Nurse A had to account for herself to an "outsider", explaining—and exposing herself to scrutiny—things she felt should be self-evident. She was also frustrated by the limitations of the therapeutic role. While she appreciated the protection of confidentiality, which meant she could speak freely, there was a wish that the therapist could act on what she was hearing—"have a word" with someone and exercise some authority to move things on. The "screen" of polite behaviour came down and the therapist was allowed in on a more lively scene—the "mess" of Nurse A's emotional turmoil.

It was at this point that a difficult idea emerged: that Nurse A's task, at this point, might be to bear her culpability for not carrying out her legal duty to try to resuscitate the patient she had been called to see. With this issue overshadowing questions raised by Nurse A about neglect, already noticed by her around the patient's death, the hospital could continue to function, even if it was in a way that was less than ideal. Also at this time, one of her (usually silent) patients said to her, "Poor Nurse A, what are they doing to you?" The realisation that her distress was noticed, not just by the therapist but also by the patients she needed and wanted to care for, provided an incentive to do her best to remain at work, maintaining a presence as a nurse who made great efforts to offer her patients comfort and personal contact, in a way that, as she said, was sensitive to "whether they are the kind of person who wants a cuddle or wants you to respect their personal space".

Discussion

I would like to be able to report that armchairs were restored to Nurse A's ward, and that conditions improved in other ways too, benefiting both the staff and the patients. This remained unknown, however, as Nurse A needed to use her sessions to think about her retirement, and to make a decision whether to appeal against the verdict of the enquiry. The work of the therapist was to remain with the material Nurse A needed to address, and to trust that her patient was using her restored capacity to think in a professional way and would take responsibility for organisational issues that were causing her concern.

The primary task of a therapist is to work with patients, and those working for in-house therapy services for staff are not exempt from the statutory rules regarding confidentiality, privacy, and respect for the therapeutic relationship. They also need to respect the organisation, which employs both them and the staff they see. Unlike private psychotherapy, the therapist is paid by a third party, and the employing organisation very reasonably expects that she will work to its advantage: reducing unnecessary expense, for example, from sickness absence, and improving performance, so that staff continue to fulfil the organisation's duty of care towards its patients. The virtuous circle is completed in the duty of the therapist to find ways of relating to senior figures in the organisation. While maintaining the privacy of individual staff, managerial consultations offered the potential to share broad insights, informed by understanding of factors that help or undermine staff in their work. Just as the private patient expects the analyst to deliver necessary home truths, in the service of insight, so representatives of the healthy organisation need to know what might be undermining staff morale and wellbeing.

As the case of Nurse A shows, the therapist can be presented with a complex picture, made up of different accounts of life in the organisation. Because of the raw nature of some of these accounts, great care needs to be taken to maintain analytic neutrality. Inevitably, there can be feelings about seeing staff who might be being bullied, or feel under pressure to provide care that seems less than ideal. As with the case of Nurse A, there might be occasions when the therapist feels uncomfortable about her own role as recipient of these confidences.

Dealing with her own distress at what she was hearing, then focusing on the "here and now" experience of her patient, allowed the therapist to use her privileged position within the institution to remain in role, and to use her "binocular vision" to penetrate through the manifest content to an unconscious meaning, which she thought the situation might hold for Nurse A.

This way of treating psychological distress centres on the importance of containing psychic "toxicity" caused by strong negative feelings, which, in Nurse A's case, might have pushed her to breach the boundary of her professional attachment to the employing organisation in a way that was unlikely to have helped anyone. The wish to discharge disturbing feelings through action can be powerfully attractive. For Nurse A, who believed she was being made a scapegoat, the temptation to become the accuser, and restore her reputation, was considerable.

Questions arising

In addition to addressing Nurse A's distress and her underlying personal issues, born of life experiences and the way she unconsciously chose to protect herself against psychological pain, it became apparent that there were factors that needed to be thought about in organisational terms, with relevance for all staff, which might have conspired to produce an unstable context for the incident that began the investigation.

1. Nurse A had begun to think about retirement from a career in which she was highly invested and which provided a sanctuary from some troubling elements in her personal life.
2. There had been bereavement of a significant family member. Nurse A may have returned from leave in some distress, but have managed to keep this hidden from her manager and colleagues, who possibly colluded with her in not knowing about her emotional trouble.
3. The strain of professional investigation exposes staff to judgement and scrutiny from a powerful body of authority (from an ego ideal and/or superego), loss of professional agency, insecurity and disruption to a work role that provides financial independence, and professional and vocational status. It could be argued that those involved in carrying out such investigations need

training in awareness of these psychological pressures on staff, as they attempt to establish the substance and detail of events. Perhaps this level of understanding should extend to the managers of staff undergoing such investigations, whether or not they are permitted to continue working.

4. When staff continue working, but in a reduced role, there is an added complication, in that the professional boundary between staff and patients can feel as though it has been eroded, resulting in increased exposure to unconscious anxieties of the kind described by Menzies Lyth (1988a[1959a]) and others (Armstrong & Rustin, 2014).

5. In addition to these personal factors, there seemed to be some organisational issues, including the impact of short-staffing and budget cuts, which put additional pressure on all the staff. The therapist wondered if the apparent silence around the removal of patients' comfortable chairs was part of the same defence against acknowledging patients' suffering as Nurse A suffered from in the course of the enquiry: silence and non-communication.

6. There was a question why Nurse A had not been able to think about her discomfort with an aspect of her job that went strongly against the grain, in a way that might have helped her to be better prepared for such a troubling situation—especially as the case of Janet Tracey was so much in the news.[8]

7. The question of how nurses on older adult wards and units are trained to cope with situations such as this one seemed not to form part of the enquiry into this incident. It is possible that the isolation and helplessness of her patients, which Nurse A worked so hard to alleviate, came uncomfortably close to anxieties about her own approaching retirement—and, of course, related thoughts about her old age and death.

8. Loneliness is a known factor in the development of mental health problems in older people. A tendency to isolation can extend to the team members working with them.

9. A further question was whether the family, who brought the complaint leading to the enquiry, might not have been helped to think differently about resuscitation of their elderly relative, given his illness and frail state. This sensitive issue, I would suggest, needs to be given careful consideration, if proposals for a state-registered older people's nurse are taken forward. As Jane

Garner, commenting on the implications for staff of the Francis Report (2014), notes:

Francis mentions that caring approaches are applicable to all but makes particular mention of the elderly, including considering the introduction of a new state-registered older person's nurse. As staff working with older patients often share their stigma, thought needs to be given to this new role so it is associated with the status afforded other specialisms. All staff need to understand life cycle changes, dependency issues in old age, the multiple nature and complexity of problems encountered in later life, the interplay between mental and physical health, restricted mobility, financial and environmental constraints, social impoverishment and isolation and ageism (which will affect society, the staff and also the patient themselves) . . . *Staff . . . may need help talking about death, their previous experience and their own anticipated end . . .* (Garner, 2014, pp. 216–217, my emphasis)

The vocational motivation and psychological vulnerability of mental health staff

This event changed Nurse A's experience of work as a place of care, in which she could offer something good to her elderly patients, into a place in which she found herself exposed to her worst fears, which could be traced back to her childhood. First, a family death, then that of a patient, followed by a public stripping of her professional authority, with her reputation, as she felt it to be, "in tatters", and, perhaps worst of all, the prolonged period of helplessness, in which she felt there was no clear information about timing and process; the cumulative effect of this experience resonated with her childhood sense of being blanked by a mother who could unexpectedly lapse into an absent, possibly fugue-like state. The therapeutic work needed to focus on her subjective experience of these events, in an attempt to heal the wound in the mind that is trauma. The aim was to help Nurse A find her own thinking mind, do herself justice during the various meetings she was called to in the course of her enquiry, and make her own decisions about whether to accept the verdict against her, or to appeal against it.

Underlying her personal narrative, it was possible for the therapist to identify some psychological issues, familiar from her work with other mental health staff, and described succinctly by Banks (2002). Writing from long experience of working with NHS staff in both medical and mental health settings, and especially drawing on an in-depth study of the personality of staff working in mental health (Banks, 1997), she identified a "constellation of personality traits in healers", which seemed to be quite pervasive:

> Chief among them are a narcissistic need for omnipotence and a struggle to resolve the Oedipal conflict. Others include an attempt to repair the damaged mother; empathy towards the wounded patients by identification; reaction formation; the attempt to master personal conflicts; the use of work and patients as a transitional object; and the dyads of sado-masochism, rescue and reparation, and power and control. (Banks, 2002, p. 23)

So long as work goes well, and is properly supported, managed, and supervised, such underlying traits might not create problems. When these conditions are not met, staff could experience a frightening level of psychological difficulty, as their unresolved issues and conflicts are exposed.

In addition to the personality and meaningful life events of the individual member of staff, there are the social defences (Menzies Lyth, 1988a[1959a]), which those working in healthcare settings need to erect in order to function in circumstances that, like trauma, can confront them with profoundly anxiety-provoking situations.

Obholzer coined a phrase to denote the way the NHS is expected to protect society from unconscious anxieties associated with death. He describes society's need to create systems that defend us all against such fears—effectively, he says, for "a health service to serve as a keep death at bay service" (Obholzer, 1994, p. 171).

With mental health problems, such survival anxieties might extend to fear of mental "infection", as Hinshelwood identified in his discussion of a series of observations of mental health settings (Hinshelwood & Skogstad, 2000). Hinshelwood identified a particular fear, which he considered to be operating on the same primary level as the death anxieties Obholzer described in medical settings: "the critical anxiety [of] someone dying . . . is not so evident in a psychiatric setting. Here, the fear is of madness. One could say that madness is a kind of death of the mind . . ." (Hinshelwood & Skogstad, 2000, p. 157).

Mental health staff are faced with such anxieties on a daily basis, countering their fear with their professional defences and also with their capacity to think about and to alleviate the suffering of their patients. As we have seen in the case of Nurse A, this capacity to care originates from deeply personal experiences. Her care for the minds, as well as the bodies, of her patients seemed to her therapist to be this nurse's way of attending to the pain and helplessness (her own? her mother's?) when she lost the containment of her mother's mind: first, she became a thoughtful, good student, then a thoughtful, good nurse and mental health nurse. When this solution was threatened, Nurse A found herself close to physical and mental breakdown.

The psychological vulnerability of mental health staff—alongside their resilience, psychological-mindedness, and resourcefulness—is an important factor to take into account when thinking about their needs. As Cooper and Lousada (2005, p. 113) remind us, "For mental health clinicians the work, if done well, disturbs the practitioner". They emphasise the need for a "psychologically sensitive environment", in order to provide the conditions for reflective practice to occur.

The scene witnessed by the therapist, through Nurse A's eyes, was the reverse of this, with staff working in a split and stratified way—two sectors of staff, literally "screened off", the one from the other. While the rigid hierarchy described by Menzies Lyth could preclude empathetic, human contact, at least it was informed by an awareness of the need for good physical nursing care, which ran through the staffing structure. Splitting off the functions of qualified nurses working on computers, and unqualified HCAs carrying out the tasks of nursing care, seemed to the therapist to be conducive to a disturbing level of blindness to all patients' needs. Sir Robert Francis, reporting on the Mid Staffs enquiry, condemned a form of care in which the patient was sacrificed to the "tick-box" requirements of a target-driven system. Such a system can be described as operating in survival mode, in a field of work in which survival anxiety is experienced as a primary threat.

As we have seen, nurses, whether working in general medical or mental health settings, are motivated by a deeply personal, vocational need to care and repair (Dartington, 2010, pp. 211–212; Roberts, 1994a). There is a danger that, if this opportunity is not provided and properly supported, the more thoughtful staff will leave, feeling undervalued and demoralised, and possibly finding agency work. Those that remain, and remain sensitive, are vulnerable: to developing "psychosomatic symptoms, the avoidance of work, long periods of sick-leave, depression and, ultimately, resignation" (Dartington, 1994, p. 107). These are the staff members who are likely to find their way to counselling services. Others might develop psychological defences against the pain of witnessing suffering they cannot relieve, protecting themselves by forming a

> shell around themselves which serves to deflect and anaesthetize emotion. This is largely an unconscious development. If such a shell becomes a permanent feature of the personality, it is at great cost to the individual, who can no longer be fully responsive to his or her emotional environment. The resulting detachment is dangerous to clients, patients or colleagues, who will sense the potential cruelty inherent in the indifference. (Dartington, 1994, p. 107)

The Francis Report made detailed recommendations, in order to support improvements in the attitudes, training, and support of both clinical and managerial staff. His emphasis on the need for compassion, echoed and amplified by representatives from all levels of society, led one commentator to wonder: "what has gone so wrong . . . that a high court judge has to write a report emphasising the need for compassion in nursing when this should be taken as a given" (Evans, 2014, p. 193). Evans's contention is that well-meaning attempts to train and monitor the way care is provided do not go far enough. Sadly, this is borne out as we continue to hear about similar abuses, not just in in-patient settings, but in other agencies that are entrusted with the work of assessing, evaluating, and meeting the needs of those who struggle to manage in the community (see Bell, 2013).

Evans identifies the unconscious impact on staff of the imperatives driving healthcare organisations:

> only exceptional clinical managers can juggle the demands between the persecution of the "target culture" while keeping the care of the patients at the heart of their thinking. . . . As Lord Francis said in his report, we need to put the clinical care and nurturing of our patients back at the heart of the NHS. In order to do so, we need to start addressing the current moralistic and persecutory culture of the current NHS. (Evans, 2014, p. 209)

The therapist working with Nurse A found herself, at the end of the day, agreeing with the character reference provided for this "good nurse", who seemed to be a casualty in a system in which, as described above, good nurses leave, feeling demoralised, devalued, and unsupported. Hard as this experience was for Nurse A, it is equally hard for the patients, those who care about them, and an NHS that, on paper at least, is crying out for better nursing care.

CHAPTER TEN

The organisational context for good care

Tim Dartington

Introduction

A few years ago, the chief executive of a mental health trust said to me, "We are not good at looking after our own." He was talking about a respected clinician, who was taking early retirement on grounds of ill health. Human Resources did all the right things to do with the mechanics of the retirement: the financial aspects, the pension arrangements. But somehow this was not enough, in his mind. So what did he mean?

I want to explore the dynamics of care to see how it might be difficult at times for those whose business is managing therapeutic interventions to show compassion towards those who are doing the work. Then I will make the argument why it is important to give greater management attention to care for the carers, and how the containment of anxiety is in danger of becoming a neglected management function. In this context, non-managerial supervision, reflective practice, even an in-house counselling service might be seen both as a necessary resource to stressed staff and a way for the system to be self-reflective. We know that working with patients, not only those diagnosed with mental illness, can easily get under the skin of clinical staff. It might, then, be appropriate to offer them psychoanalytic therapy, when the work sets off personal issues in their own lives.

My approach is both systemic and psychodynamic: that is, I see organisations as open systems, relating to their environment and providing the conditions for good work to be done. This is analogous to ways that we manage ourselves as individuals, as we manage ourselves in different roles and negotiate between our inner world of thought and fantasy that we create in our own minds from early child-hood and our adult identities exposed to the external realities we face in our everyday lives. This negotiation involves both conscious and unconscious communication between ourselves and others. There are helpful concepts, developed by psychoanalysts in their exploration of individual development, of good enough mothering, the capacity for thought, and the management of anxiety, which are applicable more generally to our relations in adult life, to our relationships at work, and have an acute relevance when the work has to do with the needs of those in physical and mental distress—working in systems of care. I am thinking, for example, of the capacity for reverie that a mother experiences in understanding her child's emotions long before the infant has the power of speech and how this allows the mother to contain the anxiety of the child, learning to live with brief separations or the frustration that arises with hunger. And how the child experiences fierce love and hate towards the same object (including the mother herself) and the containment offered by the mother then contributes to the child's capacity to tolerate these extremes of feeling. I am also thinking how we retain in our mature selves a capacity to see the world at times as black and white, good and bad, especially when we are under stress, and how we have a capacity to hate in others what we would want to reject in ourselves—for example, feelings of vulnerability. The psychoanalytic concepts of splitting and projection mean that we retain a strong tendency to see ourselves in the right and others in the wrong, which, at times, may be true but not always, and on reflection we know that it is rarely as simple as that.

In my work as a researcher and a consultant to groups and organisations in health and social care, it has been possible, with this approach, to enquire as to what are the organisational conditions conducive to developing a culture of compassion and empathy in relations with others, colleagues and patients, and what are the conditions that lead to bullying and scapegoating of colleagues and indifferent care of patients.

Anxiety in organisations working with vulnerable people

Large organisations—large enough for their members to be anony-mous to each other, unacknowledged and unexamined objects of mutual mistrust—are likely to be full of anxiety. The anxiety in the group can be described as psychotic, when it acts as if excessively threatened and fearful of the other, although individually the people in the group are sane and well balanced. Why is that? The experien-tial study of group process in Tavistock group relations conferences demonstrates time and again how readily our individual capacity for making sense may be taken over by more primitive connections being made, including our need to belong while struggling with our fear of the other. In his study of identity in the large group, Pierre Turquet (1975) distinguished between the individual member (IM), who retains a sense of autonomy, and the membership individual (MI), "where group membership predominates over individual self-defini-tion and needs, and so destroys his I.M. state".

As Otto Fenichel (1946) says, "Social institutions influence the instinctual structures of the people living under them, through temp-tations and frustrations, through shaping desires and antipathies". He was an influence on the work of Isabel Menzies Lyth (1988a,b[1959a,b]) and her influential study of social defences in nursing as a defence against anxiety.

I want to consider the implications of a psychoanalytic under-standing of anxiety, when this leads to a persecutory fear for the survival of our ego or sense of self. We are not talking only of ordi-nary fears that might be quite reasonable in the circumstances—the fear that I might lose my job, or the worry that my boss does not like me—and all the ordinary unhappinesses of day-to-day living. A colleague, with whom I was observing the work of an acute admis-sions ward in a psychiatric unit, made the common sense comment that no one gets up in the morning wanting to do a bad job. But what happens when you go to work? We may think from our own experi-ence how we adopt a state of mind when we enter a system—cautious, enthusiastic, interested, bored, fearful, curious, tired, energised, and so on. The effect of going to work might make you feel good about yourself, or you might feel depressed, resentful, or angry.

To be without psychological defences would be the equivalent of going out in all weathers without appropriate clothing. When we are talking about social defences, building on the work of Menzies Lyth, our concern as clinicians, managers, researchers, organisational consultants, change agents, patients, and users of services, in whatever role we find ourselves, is with those defences that are dysfunctional, that get in the way of doing a good job, that contribute to abusive relationships and relatedness to the vulnerable other.

Everyday fears and worries could provoke and feed on a deeper underlying anxiety, which makes our reaction more intense, beyond our control, and leads to dysfunctional outcomes. In a collection of essays on social defences, published fifty years after Menzies Lyth, several authors have described different contexts for the expression of anxiety, not only in health and social care. For example, Jon Stokes (2015) distinguishes personal and professional anxiety in the legal profession, with its predisposition to carefulness and caution and "healthy sense of mistrust"! For myself, I want to focus on anxiety provoked by uncertainties of outcome in health and social care, which then contributes to a catastrophic lack of meaning—an existential crisis, where we lose touch with the purpose of what we are doing.

Anxiety is a word in such common use, and so ill defined (generally speaking, not defined at all) that our discourse suffers as a result. It brings forth subjectively unpleasant feelings of dread over anticipated events, including feelings of annihilation. Anxiety is not the same as fear, a response to a real or perceived immediate threat, but is the expectation of future threat, and may be identified as an overreaction, objectively speaking, to a situation that is subjectively seen as menacing.

Existential anxiety was described by the theologian Paul Tillich (1952, p. 44) as "the state in which a being is aware of its possible nonbeing". What, for some, would be a spiritual exercise is, for others, a fear of annihilation, following a loss of meaning and purpose. Tillich argues that this anxiety can be accepted as part of the human condition or it can be resisted, but with negative consequences. In its pathological form, it may "drive the person toward the creation of certitude in systems of meaning which are supported by tradition and authority". So, anxiety pushes us towards certainties that are not justified, the other side of the coin to living with not knowing, negative capability, as described by the poet John Keats: "when man is capable of being in uncertainties, mysteries, doubts, without any irritable reaching after fact and reason" (Keats, 1970[1817], p. 43; French, 2001).

In her study of social defences in nursing, Menzies Lyth drew attention to the stress of the work: nursing tasks that are distasteful, disgusting, and frightening, or arousing libidinal and erotic wishes and impulses difficult to control. She saw a striking resemblance then to unconscious phantasy situations in the deepest and most primitive levels of the mind, life and death instincts at work below the surface of everyday behaviour. This is when stress might provoke anxiety in the nurse and lead to dysfunctional responses to the nursing task.

I emphasise again, as she did, that psychological defences are essential to our everyday living. In order to focus on one thing, we have to exclude others, in the way that we close the door when we need to concentrate or want privacy; this becomes problematic only when we want to keep the door closed or locked. In the same way, we think of boundaries as healthy mechanisms, except that we have to remember that boundaries are meant to be permeable. The skill in human interaction comes from managing the transactions across boundaries. It is when we observe dysfunctional outcomes of defensive behaviour that we need to investigate further: the defensive behaviour gives us a clue to something unhealthy that is going on in the system. The existential crisis of feeling stressed in a way that is out of control—being unable to do a good job, unappreciated for the effort one is making, a feeling of being unloved and invisible, leading to a loss of faith in what one is doing—might provoke, for example, a paranoid–schizoid response, leading to bullying of colleagues and conscious or unconscious cruelty towards patients, defending an embattled sense of self at the expense of empathy for the other.

Our professional identities act as defensive systems against anxiety; that is, they protect us from crippling self-doubt. There is an underlying lack of self-confidence even in the high-achieving individual—this becomes apparent, for example, when such a person loses their job—and the job insecurity of high-flying individuals may, in fact, be a considerable threat to their identity. The chief executives of NHS Trusts are under great pressure to perform, experiencing a heady mix of political and economic demands. This insecurity at the top is epitomised by the insecurity of politicians uneasily aware that the next cabinet reshuffle or general election might cast them into the outer darkness. It is surely contributory to the culture of bullying and intimidation, and the persecution of whistleblowers, that can be observed in public sector organisations financed from general taxation and subject to intense political scrutiny. Private sector organisations are not exempt from these pressures, as their contracts are also constrained by narrowly defined value for money arguments.

Our society has shifted radically within our lifetimes from a general acceptance of the dependability and continuity of institutions, which, for very many people, meant a "job for life", to an increasingly uncertain culture of manic reorganisation, merger, and collapse, within short time-frames (Khaleelee & Miller, 1985). It is arguable that, in this post-dependent world, we live in a punitive society, where failure is punished like a sin, leading to the fear of being excluded, cast out, rather than learning and recovery. Where there is a breakdown of containment, of the capacity to tolerate and detoxify the pain of others, we might see the development of a second skin, less permeable than the first and insensitive to nuances of feeling.

The societal context of organisational defences in health and social care

Human service organisations are always going to be defensive against the possibility of overwhelming need. In our interactions with others, in our personal and professional relationships, we put limits on what we are prepared to do. When there is always the possibility that we could do more, we work hard to maintain a good enough identity, so that we may feel good about ourselves and not be incapacitated by guilt and doubt and depressive anxiety.

Menzies Lyth described how disturbing emotions to do with death and sexuality might arise in nurses, especially students. But nurses develop their defensive behaviours in the context of wider societal projections of a fearful and even threatening dependency in those who are vulnerable: people with disabilities, those with long-term conditions, the old and the dying.

We might think also how the vulnerability of others leads to their dehumanising in the public imagination, associated with moral panic and paranoid anxiety towards those such as asylum seekers (includ-

ing children), prisoners (including the mentally ill), and other populations whose humanitarian needs must be denied if they are to be
feared and hated without remorse, leading to the probability of institutionalised neglect and cruelty.

When we talk of front-line staff, we are using a military metaphor.
Is it so fanciful to think of customers (or patients) as the enemy? When
we describe the more vulnerable people in society as sick, as patients,
as having special needs, this is an attempt to detoxify their dependency. This is one reason why it might be helpful to patients to have
a diagnosis (even if this is fearful, as, for example, in the diagnosis of
dementia), if this helps to legitimise their need. But they are also challenging our own sense of identity by behaving differently towards us,
by making demands simply by being there, and this puts them at risk
of our unconscious retribution. The system of care, which is intended
to be responsive and compassionate, becomes itself a receptacle for
our own unwanted projections of inadequacy into others.

Compassion, running counter to this dynamic, is intrinsic to care
and to nursing tasks fundamental to this purpose, and it is question-
able whether this is a taught competence. The Willis Commission on
Nursing Education (2012) drew attention to the importance of personal mentoring for students and, at the same time, the pressures on
this resource, restricting its effectiveness.

Some current management practices undermine the autonomy of
the care relationship of meaning through an instrumental approach
that routinises work practices. The focus is on the defensive behaviour
of those in the care relationship, the care assistant and the nurse, who
are being trained to see people as fragmented, as less than whole, so
that they are treated as a series of tasks and protocols, with an emphasis on making a record of interactions rather than keeping outcomes
in mind. The anxious behaviour of managers is one activity that goes
unrecorded in this process. To be vulnerable is to be human, but vulnerability implies a greater than normal exposure to threat or danger.
The exercise of power often involves the denial of that vulnerability in
ourselves, while, at the same time, locating and exploiting it in others.
This is the built-in bias of the care relationship, which anxious
management could exacerbate.

We have seen that stress arises naturally in any system of care. It
has to do with managing the balance between love and hate aroused
by the vulnerability of the other. If we accept that there is always

going to be stress in a system of care, then it follows that this stress is always going to be expressed in one way or another. For example, the role of receptionist is important in managing the boundary of what is outside trying to get in—in a clinic, the patients!—and the benign clinician may be protected in that role by the officious or indifferent receptionist. Automated receptionist systems are increasingly in use, institutionalising this process. Or it may work the other way, the receptionist humanising an indifferent or mechanistic service from a stressed clinician.

Efficient management may seek to compartmentalise services, each to be monitored on its own performance, and then it is as if the love and the hate in the system have to be kept separate, so that the one does not get to contaminate the other. In a more integrated systemic culture, an individual might experience both love and hate in relation to the patient, often from moment to moment, as many therapists will understand.

Social defences are, thus, not simply an individual's way of responding to stress. They become institutionalised and acculturated into ways of doing things that might be largely unexamined and unquestioned. An instrumental approach to relationships—reduced to a series of tasks—contributes to "borderline welfare", systems of care that lack the capacity to tolerate mental pain:

> the fear is that once we allow real contact with a deprived, dependent, helpless population, any services offered to them will become rapidly enslaved to their needs for all time, draining resources from other important projects, and depleting our autonomy and flexibility as a society and an economy. (Cooper & Lousada, 2005, p. 194)

There is an argument to be made instead for "intelligent kindness", a compassionate understanding of our interdependence, the kinship that is the root meaning of kindness:

> the challenge involves recognising the uncomfortable reality that the industrialisation of healthcare, the development of a competitive market and regulatory processes, however expertly or ineptly applied, will always tend to draw healthcare staff's attention away from here-and-now possibilities of effective kindness. (Ballatt & Campling, 2011, p. 172)

A difficulty with the concept of failing organisations is that we think to close them down without learning from the mistakes made. With the closure of the old asylums, we lost the continuing opportunity to make them more humane. So, again, we do not get it right, for example in care homes, which more than one commentator has argued do not care and are not home:

> When abuse and torture were exposed at Winterbourne View by the BBC Panorama programme on May 2011, all the outside bodies which, in different ways, had oversight of and responsibility for the care of the people living there, reacted by imposing more of the measures and practices that had already failed to protect the residents of Winterbourne View. Instead of examining their own core tasks in relation to care providers, they reinforced systems of regulation and review that had already failed so tragically. (Burton, 2015, p. 41)

Extreme cases of cruelty and neglect (Stafford Hospital has been a recent example) are exposed, but only with great difficulty and persistence. They are then roundly condemned, most loudly by those who contribute to the conditions that made the scandals possible. Another response, much quieter, but widespread in the NHS, has been to face the near-unthinkable proposition that "it could have been us".

According to this argument, the cruelty and the unnecessary deaths exposed at Stafford are not an aberration but a near-inevitable consequence of a societal denigration of care, as evidenced by poor working conditions, inadequate staffing levels, and indifferent management preoccupied with financial targets. The costs of dependency are experienced as threatening to our economic security, and, as citizens, we come to accept the argument that we cannot afford the public services that, as families, we look for in times of need.

My hypothesis is that regulation without insight leads to bullying and to the silencing of dissent. The exposure of institutional abuse is always shocking. The public reaction is, how could that happen? The political response is, it must not happen again. The Mid-Staffordshire NHS Trust Inquiry (Francis, 2010) has been an example of the political response, the insistence that it must not happen again, and yet, at first, the government was reluctant to institute a public inquiry, making the argument that it was unnecessary because of the system of regulation that was in place.

Whistleblowers experience the personal cost of speaking truth to power, as they find themselves ignored, intimidated, or worse. They can expect unsympathetic treatment themselves, because they are subversive and disruptive to a hierarchical authority determined to manage and keep under control the emotional content of the work. The trouble with emotion at work is that it is difficult to manage.

Many examples of failure of care are linked to resource management, low levels of staff, and inadequate training and supervision. From this perspective, it is as if clinical staff members are being asked to make bricks without straw and then are held accountable when the service collapses. Front-line staff are more likely to face suspension and dismissal for failures of care than senior managers, who are more at risk from the failure to meet financial targets.

Publicly funded services are required to make efficiency savings. Private sector services are commissioned to provide services at the lowest cost. Compassionate care is not always efficient from this perspective. I have described, in an earlier study of the inter-agency relations to do with services for the elderly mentally infirm, how intractable problems associated with dependency in old age were too much for one agency to take on as its primary activity, but that a collective effort was being attempted by different agencies, for whom this was not their primary task but an associated task, and it was necessary that within each agency there were those for whom this was their chosen primary focus. This allowed those committed to doing this work to follow their own professional instincts in responding to need, and this led me to consider how some collaboration is deviant at a systemic level, challenging narrowly defined criteria for accessing resources, but essential at the emotive practitioner level. We see then how the management of resources, including resources of time, comes into conflict with a professional response to need (Dartington, 1986).

Despite a rhetoric of integration over many years, austerity policies in more recent times have seen a dramatic contraction in the provision of social care. Local leadership is as important as leadership at the top. This is the leadership that develops and sustains what we may think of as a mini-society of compassionate values, on a ward, in a clinic, or a team or agency, which is resistant to wider societal projections of lack of worth.

We might be aware of such pockets of exceptional practice. I saw one example when a family member was very ill and supported by a "package" of care at home. The carer from the local authority worked in an integrated way with the informal carers (and with occasional friction with other professionals), adapting her schedule to meet the needs of the family, alongside those of an elderly client living alone two streets away, and also those of another woman, who was disabled and had a son with learning difficulties. When our family member died, this young man gave us a rose bush from the parks department, where he worked, although he had never met us. Such relatedness could be as effective as actual relationships. Such a mini-society is easily created, but it does not sit easily with bureaucratic norms and I rather doubt whether some of the actions of the care worker would have had the approval of her managers. But such schemes may be encouraged, and the Buurtzorg ("neighbourhood care") model in the Netherlands of a nurse-led service has shown what can be done. However, a shift from command and control to an enabling culture is not so easy when services are under-funded.

Responding to suffering and the need for reflective practice

When I was a child and we were walking to church on a Sunday, I developed an acute pain in my side. The next week the same thing happened, and my mother suspected that I was trying it on to avoid going to church. Then she saw me at home: I did not know she was watching, but I had doubled over with the pain. She knew then it was for real and I was taken to hospital and the trouble was investigated. I remember this incident because it reminds me that we are often suspicious of the needs of others. Are they exaggerating? Are they really suffering? Are they avoiding their responsibilities or exploiting the system?

A lot of systemic responses to need are cautious, defensive, or suspicious and it is probably inevitable that some people are trying it on. However, it is also true that people in need do not benefit from not being believed, or being told explicitly or implicitly that the problems they have are their own fault.

Care is predicated on the assumption that people should get better. When someone in my family was in the late stages of dementia and close to death, a carer said how she was praying for her recovery. At the time it seemed a shocking denial of reality. When someone is dying, it is usual practice to admit him or her to hospital. According to recent statistics, fifty-three per cent of people die in hospital, though two-thirds of people, when surveyed, expressed the wish to die at home. While in hospital, it is implicit that every attempt be made to keep them alive as long as possible. We might think that this is a "medical model", scientific and instrumental, but here are the thoughts of two doctors on the limitations of their expertise.

Atul Gawande is a surgeon and public health researcher:

> The waning days of our lives are given over to treatments that addle our brains and sap our bodies for a sliver's chance of benefit. They are spent in institutions—nursing homes and intensive care units—where regimented, anonymous routines cut us off from all the things that matter to us in life. Our reluctance to honestly examine the experience of ageing and dying has increased the harm we inflict on people and denied them the basic comforts they most need. Lacking a coherent view of how people might live successfully all the way to their very end, we have allowed our fates to be controlled by the imperatives of medicine, technology and strangers. (Gawande, 2014, p. 9)

Henry Marsh is a neurosurgeon who emphasises, not the extra-ordinary technical skill, which is magical to the lay person, but the even more difficult work of making a judgement, and he addresses the commonplace example of resuscitation:

> The reality of cardio-pulmonary resuscitation is very different from what is shown on TV. Most attempts are miserable, violent affairs, and can involve breaking the ribs of elderly patients who would be better left to die in peace. (Marsh, 2014, p. 83)

My proposition is that care that is predicated on the denial of death is never going to be satisfactory. If a health service is primarily a "keep death at bay" service (Obholzer, 1994), privileging survival over quality of life, it cannot be fully fit for purpose. My observation is that there has to be a creative tension between "heroic" and "stoical" responses to suffering and that it is not at all easy to integrate these responses, so that they are split off into different members of the clinical team, different agencies, different services, which are in a wary and, at times, hostile relationship. Ultimately, this underpins the chronic separation of health and social care in the delivery of services to vulnerable people.

Those working in care systems are living with this profound ambivalence about responding to the needs of others. The complexity of the task, which could be programmed like computer code into a never-ending succession of binary decisions—whether to do more or to do less, to connect or reject, to intervene or let be—goes largely unrecognised in formal management systems.

Health and social care provides a methodology for reparation, for repairing the damage associated with past experience, actual or imagined. In her work with children, Melanie Klein described how, when love takes the place of aggression, "the hostile world changes into a friendly one" (Klein, 1929). William Halton (1995), describing his support for a staff counsellor in an NHS hospital, talked about "restoration of a capacity for work".

Over the years, I have worked with a wide range of health and social care organisations, mostly in the public sector but including some not-for-profit agencies and religious organisations. In each case, the contract has been specific to their needs but, broadly speaking, we have been making a space for them to think about their work, their experience of their work, and its impact on them as individuals and collectively.

I try not to have a set way of working but to be responsive as best I can to the culture and expectations of the group I am working with. Sometimes, I will be informal and chatty and, in other circumstances, I might take a more interpretative stance. I am always trying to sense what they are looking for: how I myself feel about working with them is, I think, an indicator of how they feel about themselves and their own working relations with their clients and users of services. So, if they treat me with indifference or hostility, I become curious about the difficulties they might themselves be facing with a challenging clientele.

Quite often, I do not feel that I am doing a good job. In part, this might be true enough—we are not always as helpful as we like to think. In part, it is projection from the client system, furious perhaps at my claiming a capacity to think when their experience is of not thinking. Otherwise, they would feel overwhelmed. Actually, they feel overwhelmed already, and do not want to think, because that would only make it more painful.

Because of these projective mechanisms, it is not irrelevant how the reflective practice consultant to a work group—or counsellor to an individual—is identified as an insider or outsider to the system, and, if the consultant is identified with an external agency, how this is going to put expectations on the process. I have experienced this very clearly at times in the past when I have been working for the Tavistock Institute or the Tavistock Clinic. One client described this as being Tavistocked. Perhaps because of the mythical associations to psycho-analytic thinking, I sensed an assumption or expectation that there was a potent and even threatening revelatory process on offer.

Here are brief extracts from my observations from such reflective practice, working with hospital-based teams in an NHS Trust.

Group A: Our meeting is some distance from the clinical area. The manager got there early to move the heavy table in the meeting room. We were joined by a consultant psychiatrist, two registrars, one white and one Asian, two nurses, male and female. I thought, the team looks balanced, but then I heard that the nurses were competing for one permanent position, and the manager would be chairing the interview panel. The psychiatrist said that it was like the parents having to say which child was their favourite. As we discussed the implications of sibling rivalry, I heard how staff members were treated interchangeably by a senior management indifferent to their particular interests and loyal-ties. When the group got to talk about patients, the discussion was about those who attempt suicide and end up in hospital. A woman severely disabled after jumping from a bridge would probably be discharged in the next week because of her detachment, her seeming indifference to her plight being mirrored by those making decisions about her care. I made a connection: indifference towards staff, linked with indifference towards patients.

Group B: I arrived for the meeting to find the office empty. In the next few minutes, people arrived and looked surprised to see me here. The consultant psychiatrist with this team was about to go on leave. There were two male nurses, one with a plaster cast on his arm. Another nurse gave her apologies; she had an appointment with a client. Another nurse was missing "for personal reasons". The issue this team wanted to discuss was their rivalry with a community-based team, who were "tradi-tional", and full of "wasters" who were threatened by new responsibili-ties to meet targets. A nurse described how a patient had been refused admission to hospital by a busy registrar, but she had advised the carer to return with the patient at another time, and the person was now an

in-patient. They talked of building up trust in colleagues that their judge-
ments were sound, while acknowledging that there was a certain
randomness to the system. There were so many different teams, all
potentially not wanting to get involved in the treatment of a patient. In
such ways, this team saw themselves as the good guys, apparently having
the confidence to resist the pressure to defend themselves or the hospital from patients who were going to be difficult to treat and difficult to
discharge. A Band 7 nurse was angry about an incident when she had
wanted one-to-one observation of a patient but had been overruled by
the nursing management, seeking to reduce the costs of agency nursing.
I observed how, in this discussion, the management became anonymous,
obsessed with making savings, disconnected from the task of caring. The
team members were having to work very hard to maintain their self-
esteem.

An issue in the public sector is of losing confidence in the capacity
to manage. Private sector models have been introduced. Private sector
management is only better—when it is better—when it is well enough
resourced and is able to work to its advantage in a profitable sector.
Its can-do attitudes do not always transfer so well to an under-
resourced public sector. Businesses fail all the time, in a way that is not
a helpful model for the public sector. The concept of failing schools
and now failing hospitals is not helpful, where dependability and
consistency are essential virtues in human services.

The people we are working with are conscious that they are struggling at times to provide any kind of acceptable service, so the excellence model is punitive. People respond with a passive, dependent
avoidance of taking their own authority. The challenge is to think
systematically how to move away from a pervasive organisational
culture of passive dependence, or, at least, not to press the wrong
buttons. (Policy debates that promote private sector good, public
sector bad messages contribute to a defensiveness in those who
hanker after clinical autonomy in their work. When working with
complex and uncertain issues of life and death, it requires a mature
response to welcome external audit and transparent accountability.)

In Menzies Lyth's time, the student drop-out rates in nursing could
be seen as an indicator that something was wrong in their training,
especially if, as she believed, it was often the better student who
dropped out. She saw them as disillusioned with the leadership of
senior nurses, who did not see a need, for example, to give attention

to the impact that the death of a patient might have on staff: "You get used to it," when a grief reaction is seen as inefficient.

In a work culture of temporary contracts, and zero hours contracts in social care, employees do not have what is dismissively described as "a job for life", as if that is self-evidently a bad thing. What they do have as a compensation for that loss of security and continuity of service is the capacity to change jobs, so that many nurses, for example, have come to prefer agency conditions of service to being employed in one organisation. There are drawbacks to this—not least the expense and the cover-up of "lastminute.com" management failings—but there are also advantages: I have seen instances of ways that good practice is communicated from one organisation to another by the nomadic working lives of competent and caring professionals.

At the societal level, there is diminished respect for the unenterprising. This again is something the politicians might think about when they respond angrily to the failures of services to meet clinical and financial targets. With their emphasis on enterprise and material achievement, they promote an aspirational identification at the expense of virtues to do with stability, consistency, continuity, patience, acceptance—which are also important in human service organisations.

Reflective practice might provide some insights into the dynamics of compassion (and its lack) in the working of a small team, and, as I have said, help to create in certain places a mini-society of compassionate care that is relational in its practice. Developing pockets of very good practice in this way could often be more effective than attempting widespread systemic reforms, which create new teams, agencies, merged and disaggregated services and continue to create conditions for splitting and projection.

Conclusion

What would be the optimal conditions for working with vulnerable people? There is no prescriptive answer to that. A safe environment, physically and psychologically, might need to be ordered and structured and also it might need to be volatile and flexible.

It might be thought counter-intuitive to argue for inequality in services for the vulnerable. Surely they are all equally entitled? So, we have become used to arguing against a postcode lottery and seek to put in place minimum standards and generally applicable targets. But then we also might want to make the argument of local autonomy, of the local service, and, ultimately, of the individual carer.

A problem with the collection of comparative data is that, while this may expose unacceptable bad practice, it implies in its general application that it will always be the case that some systems are doing well and that others are failing, where this might be true or they might just be doing different things well. Local autonomy has to mean that things will be done differently by different people in different contexts. This is inevitable in a responsive service. Do we want to work with this, or suppress it by the imposition of norms?

If we invest in a culture where you always do what you are told, we create a culture where you do not speak up about what is wrong. This creates the conditions for cognitive dissonance at work, with its associated stress and breakdown of the capacity for care.

It is useful to give careful attention to the inevitable dynamics of organisational stress, of inherent conflicts of interest between the functioning of a business and a therapeutic service: at any time, in any intervention, we may ask whose interests is this serving, while acknowledging that there is no simple answer.

Those who commission and manage services are seeking to meet need within the constraints of resources. Those delivering the service are doing the same. What we all know is that it does not always work out the way we intended. This is the crucial importance of those spaces which allow for reflection, from the most informal, at the water fountain or the canteen, or the pub when someone is leaving, or those structured occasions, coaching and non-managerial supervision and reflective practice groups, counselling, away days, CQC inspections, if we can overcome the defensiveness of our responses and acknowledge the underlying dynamics of love and hate, and the anxiety provoked by the vulnerability of others. It is always good to review practice and make changes; it is also good to accept humbly that at times we get it wrong. We need to be forgiving of ourselves as well as others, as in the end we are all vulnerable.

CHAPTER ELEVEN

General practice, mental health, and stress. Part 1: a dialogue

Marilyn Miller and Clare Gerada

> Discretion, tested by a hundred secrets
> Tact, tried in a thousand embarrassments,
> And what are more important,
> Heraclean cheerfulness and courage.
> (R. L. Stevenson on the ideal family doctor)

Introduction

In this dialogue, Marilyn Miller, a psychoanalytic psychotherapist with experience of senior management and currently a governor in an NHS mental health Foundation Trust, puts questions to Dr Clare Gerada, a leading figure in general practice, and Chair of the Royal College of General Practitioners (RCGP) between 2010 and 2013. Their dialogue refers to an organisational model, which was designed by Marilyn Miller as a way of thinking about general practice, clinically, locally, and nationally. This model is explored in more detail in Chapter Twelve, where it is followed by Marilyn Miller's commentary on the dialogue. It does, however, require a brief outline here, as it has helped to frame the questions.

The ABC Model provides a rudimentary mental map of three main professional activity spaces:

- the A system: one to one clinical practice in the GP surgery;
- the B system: activities in the locality—the domain of clinical commissioning groups (CCGs), health and well-being boards (HWBs), family and local community life, local voluntary and statutory networks, including NHS Trusts, and the local collective of GP practices. Recently, these activities are subject to Sustainability and Transformation Plans (STPs).
- the C system: national bodies with top-down reach into the consulting room—NHS England, The National Institute for Clinical Excellence (NICE), NHS Improvement, Care Quality Commission (CQC), and a plethora of other regulatory bodies, HM Treasury (who define many operational parameters of health and social care), the RCGP, British Medical Association (BMA), and national and international provider trusts and special interest groups.

An advantage of Dr Gerada's bird's-eye view, as a leader, is that the whole field of NHS disciplines (including daily, front-line clinical experience) is readily available for examination: top down, bottom up, and across. During our dialogue, some concepts and useful quotations came to mind. Some of these quotations are set in a different font and style as we go along, some are discussed in the next chapter. They are drawn from a wide range of discourses: psychoanalysis, general practice, management and organisational theory, and also the literature on postmodern culture, which analyses the social and psychological impact of global capitalism, the socio-economic system in which we live.

In work and life, the discourses to which these concepts belong co-exist untidily, more like a babel than with any kind of coherence. That reflects a complex, heterogeneous reality. As Schön points out, it is all too easy to divorce "the high ground" of professional and academic perspectives from "the swamp of real life practice" (1983, 1987).

GPs have to integrate the two. It is every GP's task to find a way, every ten minutes, within a crowded morning surgery, to match diagnostic rigour with a relevant (and rapid) response that fits the needs of the patient, current NICE guidelines, and local contracts agreed by CCGs. GPs are, after all, no longer independent clinical practitioners, or autonomous small businesses; they are tightly managed through a range of computerised, regulatory, feedback systems, nationally and locally. They also operate within a highly politicised environment, generated by perpetually changing national and local policy and operational frameworks. So, for example, Monitor—a top-level regulator—recently morphed through merger into NHS Improvement. This news, at the time of writing (May 2016, a month after the change), had not yet fully filtered down to local (B) and clinical (A) levels, and the website was out of date.

We have chosen to present this complex professional and political environment of general practice "in the raw", allowing Dr Gerada's own words to reveal the untidy co-existence of surface and depth, where "high ground" abstractions sit within the "swamp" of practice. Dr Gerada's answers reveal how tough is the struggle for GPs to survive in the current NHS environment. She herself does so by fluently linking political awareness and research findings directly into practice, while drawing on core psychoanalytic and group analytic concepts and providing impassioned leadership to her profession.

So our dialogue begins:

MM: Clare, would you introduce yourself?

CG: I am a general practitioner, at the autumn of my career. I have worked in and around the NHS since I was fourteen years old—initially as a pharmacy assistant, then as a receptionist in a GP surgery, then as a psychiatrist. Over the past twenty-eight years, I have been a GP in South London. During this time, I have also led my profession (as Chair of the RCGP) and for the past decade have provided care to two main groups of patients, those who are homeless, and doctors with mental health and/or addiction problems.

I have seen enormous changes and constant reorganisation through what I see as the magical thinking of politicians, who really believe that constant change can address the financial problems we face, or produce greater "efficiencies and effectiveness" (favourite policy change sales talk). Perhaps our politicians believe, when they get in a new post—frankly, a little like dogs marking their territory on lampposts—that they have to make their own mark, with yet another policy change. That is certainly how it feels on the receiving end anyway.

I became a doctor—a choice that was hard-wired into me from early childhood because of my idealisation of my father, himself a single-handed (immigrant) GP from Malta, brought in, as many were in the 1960s, to help the (then failing) NHS. The NHS has always been propped up by waves of immigrants serving their fellows in acts of kinship.

The NHS is, as described by Ballatt and Campling (2011, Dialogue Box 1), an embodiment of kinship and our last link to a perhaps idealised past. It is also a container for differences, bringing large swathes of individuals, many, like my father, coming from different socio-cultural, religious, and educational backgrounds, into one "large tent". The NHS does not just provide a health service, it acts also as a social unifier of these differences, and enables them to coalesce, contributing to sustaining the values of "Britishness".

Dialogue Box I: Kinship in the NHS

". . . we are concerned that so little attention has been given to understanding and promoting what we see as central to the NHS enterprise as a whole: its embodiment of kinship, and its expression, in the compassionate relationship between the skilled clinician and the patient" (Ballatt & Campling, 2011, p. 3).

My father taught me what it meant to be a good doctor—kind, caring, and a good listener. He also taught me that you had to be part of your community—essentially of your large group (B and C levels)—and that you had to give something back to that group, and that medicine was a vocation. So I was brought up with that multi-level, integrated ABC approach.

He used to take me on home visits and I witnessed, through the vista of being the "privileged" doctor's daughter, poverty and inequalities first-hand: overcrowded homes, shoeless and ragged children. I wanted to help! So already the embryonic medical-self was around—as in so many doctors. While mine is my story, it resonates with many tens of thousands of other doctors, which is why so many of us feel betrayed by the current state of the NHS.

MM: Things have changed so much since those earlier days, and you have been very involved with the mental health of general practitioners. From your own experience, what would you say are the main stressors in general practice today, and what form does this stress mostly take, how does it present? And would you say psychoanalytic thinking has any part to play in addressing GP stress?

CG: The key issue is an underlying (and sometimes not so underlying) fear. This is now the emotional driver at all organisational levels: individually in the consulting room, in the professional grapevines, in local groups and networks, or in the dreams and nightmares of policy-makers as they introduce yet another fanfared change of structure and language.

In the NHS Listening Events that we held following (though not as a result of) the Mid Staffs Inquiry, the main concern of staff in all disciplines was with fear—fear of annihilation, of naming, shaming, and blaming, of exposure. Perpetual daily anxiety was at unmanageable levels. The Francis Report (2013) looked at what was described as "catastrophic" staff and organisational behaviour, and found exactly that culture of fear that we, and others, did too, and a complete failure of all the many regulatory systems we now have (Dialogue Box 2).

Dialogue Box 2: Mid Staffordshire: The Francis Report and Fear

"Let me be clear: the care provided was totally unacceptable and a fundamental breach of the values of the NHS."
"(There existed) a culture of fear in which staff did not feel able to report concerns; a culture of secrecy in which the Trust board shut itself off from what was happening in its hospital and ignored its patients; and a culture of bullying which prevented people from doing their jobs properly." (Francis, 2013, Paras 10 & 12. Executive Summary)

The fear is twofold: first loss of a job and loss of the service given, along with fear of a loss of professionalism. And this is actually happening—GPs *are* losing their practices. A decrease in funding means that you cannot carry on providing the same quality or quantity of services. So there is a loss of staff. Then there is humiliation, coming from standards under fire, from cuts and a loss of clinical control, alongside these new "name-and-shame" policies.

Next, and much more complex, there is "existential fear", the internalised fear of the death of the NHS—bearing in mind that the NHS is, after all, a container for all of us for our fear of death (Obholzer, 1994, p. 171). So, what we are dealing with here is projective identification. I find that idea helpful, because it deepens my understanding of what all this fear everywhere in everyone is actually about. It is not only about survival personally and professionally, but at the organisational level, too, in a more general shared sense, there is a deeper feeling that human survival itself is threatened, because our fear of death is no longer contained by a shared idea of the NHS (Dialogue Box 3).

Dialogue Box 3: Fear and the Death Instinct

"(Klein) pinpointed the fear of annihilation as the primary anxiety — this is the fear of the death instinct working from within to annihilate the ego." (Hinshelwood, 1989, p. 130)

"Bion later linked the inability to deflect fear with a failure of the container–contained relationship." (Hinshelwood, 1989, p. 244)

MM: So you are describing a failure of the "container–contained" relationship in the current environment at all levels—clinically, locally, and in terms of the whole NHS system—with all that that implies. As if the NHS has become a massive, amplifying, echo chamber of shared fear, instead of a containing and facilitating environment, offering a sense of safety and belonging.

CG: Exactly, because staff are also then defending themselves from being shamed by projecting their own feelings of shame on to both the feared other—the "object" being the NHS itself and "out of touch" politicians. So, we then find ourselves in a persecuting spiral of fear, driving fear, driving shame, being projected back on to those who are creating the very policies that are setting off the fear—a spiral that ends in a dynamic of absolutely deadening splitting, and concrete thinking (clinicians *vs.* managers, doctors *vs.* nurses, GPs *vs.* hospital consultants and more), as we all try to survive in this toxic waste land.

We simply cannot of course.

The end result is a resort to unhealthy defences—taking sick leave, emigrating, early retirement, or the end points of splitting: whistle-blowing, bullying, a massive rise in peripatetic and agency staff. We see the end point of organisational chaos and, as now, the escalation of both calamities and costs.

MM: Menzies Lyth (1988b[1959b]) described those same behaviours in nurses—in a nursing hierarchy driven by fear and paranoid anxiety. Given such primitive anxieties, what do we know about the personal motivations in medicine for individual GPs choosing to go into general practice?

CG: Medical students, on qualification, do not tend to see general practice as a career choice—certainly not immediately, that is. For many young doctors, their urgent need after a long and often gruelling training, preceded by years of study, is to be able to demonstrate visibly their newly acquired (now metaphorical) white coat. Many choose, therefore, specialities where they can prod, and poke, and cut, and perform (outwardly) heroic tasks—so anaesthesia, emergency medicine, surgery, and medicine are chosen over the less glamorous specialities such as general practice, public health, and psychiatry. However, general practice offers much flexibility as a career choice (often welcomed by parents and carers) and provides the chance to work in a wide and interesting range of roles—from clinical to management, research and development, medical politics, and so on.

There are also unconscious motives why a newly qualified doctor might choose their speciality. The choice might be influenced by the unconscious wish to repair previous wounds: the child who experienced the loss or abuse of a sibling might chose paediatrics, the son of an alcoholic father enter the field of addiction, or, as with myself, my idealisation of, and identification with, my GP father led me, inevitably, to general practice.

As with many doctors, but possibly especially so with GPs, the desire to enter the speciality is driven by an altruistic drive to serve others. However, this desire to serve is now in constant conflict with the punitive, and changing, environment in which GPs work, which causes distress. Instead of removing themselves from the cause of the distress (in this case the toxic environment), GPs often try to mitigate against it, usually by working harder.

Some GPs are, however, faced with a series of paradoxes that disturb the match between their deeper motivations and the job they now have to do. For example:

Paradox 1—To be good doctors, we GPs need to be empathic and attuned to the suffering of our patients; yet, to survive as doctors, we need to be able to distance ourselves from our patients, putting our own oxygen mask on first.

Paradox 2—Doctors have high levels of self-criticism and believe that to be good doctors they must make their patients their first concern. They must work hard, be unselfish and altruistic, yet all of these attributes are associated with overwork, a denial of vulnerability, and a risk of depression/burnout.

Paradox 3—Many doctors feel they must be "perfect". Then they can overcome their deep-rooted self-doubt about themselves—that they are "not good enough". Yet, patients rarely follow the text-book examples of disease, hence perfectionism is never achievable, and the drive to be perfect actually leads to doctors delivering worse care through over-treatment, constant checking, and over-adherence to clinical guidelines. Closely aligned to that perfectionism is the fear of failure that has been increased recently, by the new NHS culture: both drive each other.

A large part of my practice is dealing with these stress-related GP behaviours. Let me give you an example from a GP's early years of hospital experience.

Jane was a junior doctor, only in the second year of her career. She had always done well at school—been head girl, getting straight As at GCSE and A level, and sailing through medical school. She was currently working on a surgical ward. Her first-year job was enjoyable but now she was finding her second job very tough. Due to cut-backs, she often found herself alone, caring for a ward of around twenty patients, many of them straight from theatre and very unwell. She was struggling to keep up with the paperwork and to find time to check all the patients' results, and get patients ready clerked for theatre, in the way that she knew her consultants wanted. She came in earlier and earlier for each shift, and found herself staying well beyond when she was meant to go home. She was finding herself increasingly anxious that she was not giving her all to her patients, and that she must be missing something, and was checking herself more and more. She didn't know what to do—she felt a failure, a fraud, and a terrible doctor.

So:

Paradox 4—Making our patients our first concern must not mean denying our own needs. It is this final paradox that doctors find most difficult to come to terms with. More adaptive behaviour for Jane would have been to acknowledge that the job she was being asked to do was unreasonable and that she needed to seek help at an earlier stage. But the built-in denial in doctors of their vulnerability, together with the overwhelming need to care (above all odds), meant that she, and many thousands of doctors, just kept going, risking poorer patient care due to burnout, depression, or anxiety.

There are actual death risks here: either to the patient, or to the doctor, who can die a kind of psychological death while trying to keep going in impossible circumstances, and there are, of course, actual suicides.

MM: Thinking now about this "match" between personal motivation and actual GP tasks as defined at policy and organisational levels (B and C), is there still a good-enough fit between those personal motivations for career choice, and the organisational tasks GPs are now required to do, locally and nationally, in the "new NHS"? For example, how are CCGs (publicised as a GP-led and -managed local B level system) actually working out for GPs?

CG: Ahead of the election in 2010, we were offered no more "top-down reorganisation". Then the 2012 Health and Social Care Act was brought in, ostensibly to "liberate" the NHS and put GPs in charge of commissioning (buying) specific healthcare services at the local level, as well as providing it themselves.

The Act promised to rid the NHS of bureaucratic controls and top-down management. In fact, the very opposite happened . . . we got the biggest re- or dis-organisation in the history of the NHS—so large that the then Chief Executive said he could "see it from outer space". Everything was destroyed. I argued at the time what the government was doing was dismantling a stately home—an old, precious building that was in good-enough repair (could do better but . . .)—and rebuilding it, but this time without windows, doors, or some of the cornerstone foundations needed for any building to continue to stand.

As we all know, admissions to hospital are now, for good reasons, kept as brief as possible and GPs shoulder the burden of clinical work being transferred out of hospital totally, or at an earlier stage of treatment, without a simultaneous shift of resources—so we now undertake ninety per cent of all healthcare activity for less than eight per cent of the NHS budget. Many in policy areas feel that GPs should now be aiming for ten per cent of the budget, because we are expected to do now what only ten years ago would have been managed entirely in hospital, and by specialists with a team of others at their elbows 24/7, and under their own leadership.

I could talk much more about the demands on general practice—the current demoralisation and death by a thousand cuts. We had the "Liberation" agenda, and before that the "Primary Care Led NHS": neither have come to fruition. Instead, GPs are treated as factory workers, having to be managed and directed by others.

GPs are now caught up in this production-line model—the industry of healthcare. Patients become depersonalised, dehumanised into "aliquots of health activity", and GPs are reduced to working on the conveyor belt. GPs actually need to have their fingers first and fore-most on the public's pulse, not the public purse. The changes to language in healthcare, and the creation of a two-tier class system, is akin to the low-cost air industry—but with the risk of leaving the poor and the vulnerable behind on the tarmac.

MM: The production-line model, with its focus on time, activity, and money—squeezing more out of each GP—also means that patients are being looked at as things rather than people ... your use of this striking phrase "aliquots of health activity" seems to exemplify this "thing-thinking" ... but it is part of an archaic industrial model, Taylorism, whose limitations have long been well-known (Dialogue Box 4).

Dialogue Box 4: Taylorism: Time and Motion—workers as extensions of machines

"In Taylor's view, the task of ... management ... was to determine the best way for the worker to do the job, to provide the proper tools and training and to provide incentives for good performance. [He] broke down each job into its individual motions, analysed these to determine which were essential, and timed the workers with a stopwatch. With unnecessary motion eliminated, the worker, follow-ing a machine-like route, became far more productive." (Taylor, 1911, p. 54)

Compare the NHS Agenda for Change of 2005:

". . . a framework for pay grades and career development [was established] ... In the attempt to create equity, [staff] had to account for every hour of their time using diaries and fit the prescribed activ-ity into bureaucratic categories. Prior to this, the informal under-standing was that they were paid to do their appointed job with whatever it took in terms of extra hours." (Ballatt & Campling, 2011, p. 146)

MM: Clare, you are referring to a depersonalisation of healthcare that is happening, but I have in mind here that the word "familiar" is related to the word "family" ... and that GPs are sometimes called "family" or "personal" doctors; also that rapid change "defamiliarises" everything. Given the increas-ingly global market of healthcare that has been developed in the past twenty-five years, and the way that it now functions, have GPs lost (or are they losing) their professional identity and role as "family doctors", "personal doctors", with a fair degree of clinical and managerial autonomy?

CG: In the modern NHS, GPs are not only family doctors, they now have multiple roles: clinician, family doctor, teacher, commissioner, public health expert, rationer of care, and, inevitably, politician. We have suffered professionally over the past few years. Promised central stage in the new NHS, we are now reduced to fighting for survival, defending ourselves against excessive and unjust criticism from politicians and the press and trying to maintain a modicum of normality against intolerable pressures.

GPs are currently being treated as the deviant part of the NHS workforce—accused by out-of-touch politicians of not pulling their weight, and needing to work harder. This is despite the fact that we are already working flat-out trying to deliver care, and provide information on what we do. We are too often being placed in the role of the naughty child—one that shows potential, but never actually delivers.

In some ways, GPs have taken over the scapegoat role of social workers in current social consciousness. Our professional identity is being challenged on all fronts—politicians demanding more for less, the media accusing us of being lazy and overpaid, patients blaming us for not being there when needed, and hospital doctors who blame us for not doing enough to keep patients out of hospital.

So, it is hardly surprising that more and more GPs are leaving the profession early, and that the training places of the next generation remain unfilled. They feel abandoned by the system they once loved, and that once loved them. Some GPs whom I see in my "sick doctor" service, and others who attend my practitioner therapy groups, describe the NHS as turning from a providing, containing, and nurturing "environmental mother" into a failing and persecutory parent, and leaving them, GPs, as helpless abused orphans. Instead of tackling the system itself (and the over-demanding and punitive masters of that system), and responding to the changes in a rational (adult) way, GPs are giving up, acting out, or becoming helpless victims, giving more and more to their patients and the NHS. This is a maladaptive way of coping with stress. Rather like the battered wife or child, they accept and absorb rather helplessly the voices of their critics, and try harder and harder to please—staying later, working harder, trying to create small miracles. Somewhere along the line, again akin to the battered child, they feel to blame for their predicament, and that they must make it good even if this is impossible.

Gerhard Wilke talks of general practice as being "currently in a mid-life crisis" and says that each person working within it has to do the psychological work necessary to find a way of surviving the transition (Wilke et al., 2000). All in the NHS have to do the work of mourning their past (idealised or otherwise), and their place in the old order, and face what it is in the new one: medicine, politics, and management.

The new order includes the move to an appointments system that operates on a basis of "any time, any place, any one"—what I call "taxi-rank general practice"—removing the time-honoured and effective concept of continuity of care, which is the cornerstone of family medicine. Continuity works for the patient and the doctor. It improves outcome, improves satisfaction, and lowers cost. But this does not sit easily with the 24/7 culture demanded largely from the fit, the well, and the young, and with it the denigration of the dyadic relationship. Instead, we are moving to "matrix care". So, the doctor–patient relationship is now located in a network—the nodal points being the computer and the electronic patient record.

This is moving right away from personalised care.

In the end, however, the basic art of caring has not changed—the interaction between patient and doctor, in the privacy of the consulting room—dealing with the physical, psychological, and, increasingly, spiritual needs of the patient. Dealing with over a million patients per day, in London, GPs see 10,000 children per hour. We also deal, as ever, with undifferentiated adult problems ("tired all the time", "pain all over"). This hasn't changed.

Policymakers and health economists might aim, misguidedly in my view, to industrialise health care, but the basic needs of the patient—for "a doctor who listens, a doctor who is there and a doctor who knows what to do"—remains constant despite the current craze for commodification and measurement. I believe the sacred relationship between the doctor and patient must be protected, but it is certainly at risk.

In this process of industrialisation—everything has its price, and nothing a value—GP services are being measured and weighed. We have moved healthcare into the factory production line in the mistaken belief that treating the sick is akin to building cars.

Perhaps, in the mental health sphere, the best example of this industrialisation of care is within the "talking therapies" and the improving access to psychological therapies (IAPT) policy. Brought in for the best of reasons—as the name suggests—this policy has instead become a production line, standardised, dumbing down of the art of medicine. Talking and listening (be it through a behavioural, cognitive, psychoanalytic, or other modality) has been reduced to treatment that is akin to a drive-in, drive-out, "Kwikfit" psychotherapy. Of course, if well-trained, the therapist can improve the mental health and well-being of the patient, but the drive for targets, and rapid throughput, with fixed and often arbitrary quantities of therapy available, and with computer feedback sheets before and after every session, is stripping out the human aspects of therapy.

Of course, GPs can manage change, nothing ever stands still, and GPs, and therapists, can adapt. But, in adapting, we are in a new, unfamiliar world where the past can give no prediction for the future—we are all in a state of permanent flux, having to relearn, and re-create, the future on the hoof—before the future becomes dismantled for yet another new future, yet another set of acronyms. The skills we need going forward, therefore, are those of survival—how to create new relationships, survive constant organisational turmoil, speak in many tongues—find *internal good* rather than expect it to be given to us from outside.

MM: It is almost Darwinian, the struggle for survival you are describing here. Jameson (1991) makes that very point: he says we have been unable to evolve quickly enough to keep up with these "high tech" market systems that define public life now.

CG: When change is too much, and too rapid, and too deep, it destabilises the complex eco-system that is the NHS—leaving us unable to recover, or adapt, to regain the capacity to care for others (or indeed ourselves). That is what we now are now witnessing.

MM: Part of this picture is that health information, and advice, has been increasingly democratised through the internet. Do we need a total rethink about the organisational frameworks for, and indeed the very nature of, general practice?

CG: There is a great deal of research around the internet and general practice and also around the internet and groups. In my view, the internet—and its educational use by patients to understand their illnesses—will increase rather than decrease the need for a generalist to translate what they find and learn. That has been my experience.

An experienced GP, who knows his or her patients over many years, can use the ten minutes per patient very effectively. They develop a sixth sense of reading the body the moment the patient walks in the room, and placing it in the context of what they already know of that patient. Intuition also becomes more finely attuned over the years, so assessing the new, and knowing when to investigate further and when not, when to pause for thought and arrange to see the patient again, comes more naturally. No internet search can compete with the kind of experienced knowhow that is general practice.

I love general practice and believe in it. I am distraught at watching it change beyond recognition, and seeing every day the many ways its survival is now threatened.

Dialogue Box 5: Commodification of Professional Services

"Commodifying the work of professionals has undermined the intrinsic value, satisfaction and enjoyment of that work, and threatens dangerously to undermine the concept of vocation to serve. For patients, always searching for signs that the professional really cares, this is bad news." (Ballatt & Campling, 2011, p. 146)

MM: Michael and Enid Balint were influential psychoanalytic voices in general practice for many years from the 1950s onwards. We used to think of doctor and patient, meeting around a presenting problem, and trying to understand it deeply. The "flash technique" and "long sessions" (M. Balint, 1955; E. Balint, 1973) of Balint-trained GPs were renowned as a creative application of psychoanalysis to general practice. The need for human-to-human storytelling was considered not only legitimate, but also a vital part of each GP's bio-psycho-social clinical assessment.

What has happened in the "new world" of general practice to the work of Michael and Enid Balint? Does this work still have a place? Is it still relevant?

CG: The Balint model was used during the golden years of both the NHS and our profession—the 1950s to the early 1990s: the period before the introduction of the NHS market. The baby-boomers were coming of age, socialist ideals were still embedded within the fabric of our society, and general practice was developing as a discipline with its own training, curriculum, examination, standards, and so on. No longer the second-class speciality, it was flourishing under the leadership of enlightened practitioners—some of whom were in Michael and Enid Balint's original groups, and founded the Royal College of General Practitioners.

Balint groups were staple fodder then for all GP trainers, and for many established GPs. I still am part of such a group today, meeting monthly. They are also a requirement in psychiatric training. The Balint model is, however, linked to that idealised NHS past I referred to earlier, where the doctor–patient relationship, and the role of the GP, was sacred, where GPs were clinicians, carers, and community leaders, all at the same time, as I have been myself for most of my career, working and living in the same place for thirty years. But this is all changing, has changed, will continue to change.

Balint assumed a long-term relationship between doctor and patient, where the doctor becomes a kind of transitional object for the patient, where the doctor really knows the patient, and *vice versa*. Time existed, for some patients anyway. The GP knew the patient in the context of their wider family and social network, and to a certain extent the doctor and patient shared the same bio-psycho-social foundation matrix that Foulkes talked about (1973). However, as the population became more mobile—because patients, and GPs, live more transient lives—the GP has become more focused on access: depth is lost, and the "taxi-rank" model comes into being. The concept of "knowing the other" is fast receding into that rose-tinted past.

Furthermore, outside the training environment, few GPs can now spare the time to be part of a Balint Group. Their loss means that there is now nowhere GPs can use as a container for anxiety, and so, often, it is projected back on to the patient, who might then become a "heart-sink", or get referred on, or, just as bad, the anxiety becomes inter-nalised and emerges as depression and burnout. Even where reflective practice groups continue, the focus is no longer on the doctor–patient relationship; rather, it is on technical diagnostic issues—"what is the matter, how should it be treated?"—not, as once, the important, deeper questions of "why?" and "why now?" and "what does this mean?". However, despite the pressure, GPs do still aim to address the physical, psychological, and social aspects of the patient in every consultation.

Let me give you another example:

Anne came in with her three-year-old daughter, Kate. Anne looked concerned. Kate ran straight to the toys in the consulting room, and began to play. The first important skill of the GP is, like that of the psychoanalyst, *observation*. Anne began to explain why she was there. She was concerned that Kate had an underlying chest problem, and, despite (repeated) attendance at both the Accident and Emergency department and at the GP surgery, she was sure we were missing something. She mentioned wanting a blood test on her daughter. I listened (second important GP skill: *listen empathically*). As she talked, I felt sad and slightly perplexed (next skill: reflect/feel what is going on, use transference/countertransference).

This was a well child, yet Mum was clearly concerned, and sad, and was transmitting this to me. I sat forward, narrowed the gap between Anne and myself, and asked, "What are you worried about?" She looked at me . . . there was a moment's silence, even the little girl had stopped playing and had returned to her mother's side. I noticed a tear in her eye. I waited (GP skill number three, *silence is a diagnostic tool*). Then Anne told me she was worried her daughter was going to die. She had had a still-birth years ago—in fact the baby would have been five years old. She was sure something was wrong with Kate, just as it had been with her first daughter, five years ago. The consultation then became one of dealing with her projected health anxiety.

So, a GP's skill in building a story is about being able to use all of our senses to determine what is wrong with the patient, and, as in this example, to use our technical skill to determine who really is the patient, and what is the presenting problem. Balint groups help us focus on this doctor–patient relationship without cluttering this with details from the doctor's own personal (or indeed professional) life.

Things have changed a lot, however. So traumatising is the current NHS, that, as Wilke has pointed out, you cannot ignore the organisational self, and how this impacts on the doctor–patient relationship. Take, for example, this vignette of Anne and Kate. Imagine that the scenario also included this being the twentieth ten-minute patient of the morning, that I was running ninety minutes late, that I was by now hungry, tired, and slightly angry at the futility of some aspects of the job. Then, that Anne, too, was already irritable at being kept waiting for her daughter's appointment, and Kate was herself hungry and tired. Add into the pot an interruption or two (harassed receptionists needing prescriptions signed to meet the pharmacy deadline, and an urgent phone call needing to be taken, unfortunately during this consultation). Then, add the prospect of home visits stacking up at reception, prescriptions still to do, important results, and letters still to read. Instead of being able to notice the "other", instead of being able to attune to both Anne and Kate in the consulting room, I could easily have acquiesced to a blood test and referred Kate for a specialist opinion, terminating the consultation as quickly as possible.

To give fully to patients requires time and mental space, uncluttered by distractions or psychological impediments such as tiredness, hunger, or the deep fear that is now everywhere, as I described at the beginning. Presenting this case to a Balint group (if one had the time) could well have missed important cues about the organisational details of our mutually stressed transference and countertransference. Instead, the focus might have been almost exclusively on my personal discomfort, and my feeling unable to do the face-to-face job properly. In other words, Balint worked at level A only—a purely clinical focus, nothing about pressures on resources, or intrusive locality or national policy—the B and C levels of your Model.

Now, as Wilke calls it "Beyond Balint", we must put the needs and feelings of the GP (which was Balint's emphasis) alongside the demands of the patient, and of the NHS, as both a local and a national system (Wilke, 2005). The reflective space, the perspective, has to be expanded to include, not just doctor–patient issues, but these other interfaces and interactions too, such as between the GP and the NHS (at levels B and C); otherwise one becomes overwhelmed (quite unconsciously) by that organisational self, instead of giving it the same kind of attention and thought that we readily give to the clinical self.

Dialogue Box 6: Loss of a Capacity for Perspective

". . . Distance has been abolished . . . we are submerged and our postmodern bodies are bereft of spatial co-ordinates and practically (let alone theoretically) incapable of distanciation; meanwhile . . . the prodigious new expansion of multinational capital ends up penetrating and colonising these precapitalist enclaves." (Jameson, 1991, p. 48)

MM: You seem to be saying a kind of "zoom lens" is now required in the GP's mind, which can home in on, but also keep separated, all three ABC levels, to preserve a realistic perspective—and that is not easy to do.

So does depth listening, and this human "story-telling" time that you have illustrated, continue to have a place in the new world of general practice, or must it now be hived off to counselling, computer chat rooms, creative writing workshops, or the gym? Does its erosion account in part for the exit from general practice of so many highly trained people?

CG: What a question, it makes me sad even to start to answer it. There is only one unique tool that GPs use over and above others and that is continuity of care. With continuity inevitably come the stories patients tell us, which we build together over time, in the context of their physical, psychological, and social self, their families, environments, and sub-culture, and these stories will continue to come,

That is the main problem we have in medicine at the moment— assuming that the individual has needs that can be dealt with by computers. As if all we are now is a series of computer-stored biomedical markers, apparently with the assumption that if these measures are audited, re-measured, and amended (as they are), the individual will be OK.

Of course, this is nonsense.

People are more than the sum of their parts. We are complex individuals. We know that illness behaviour is different in different societies, and across different people, and that how we handle adversity is also highly personal. Assuming that we can miss out the storytelling, and reduce care to the machine-marked care indices of today, misses the point entirely. Storytelling is part and parcel of what the GP–patient relationship should do—over generations. It's why I can determine whether someone is ill or not within seconds of their arrival: because I know their story already. Everything else maps on to this.

This question is so important that if there were word space I would talk about how GPs are able to do their job so well—within seconds or a few minutes. My head is full of patient stories and this is why I am a good GP. I hold so much information about patients, and it is this information that means I can use the space between me and them— the unconscious space—to determine each time what might be going on, what might be wrong. It is this space where the diagnostic acumen of the GP becomes so important.

Without the patient's story, I become an Uber rather than a black-cab doctor. I still know where to take the patient, but I have to rely, metaphorically speaking, on "sat-nav technology" to get me there, not my depth of knowledge built up over years of the different routes, side roads, back streets, and so on. Nothing can replace that lived experience.

MM: There has been a policy shift toward managing single episodes of "illness presentation" and seeking this rapid "tick-box" closure in a measured and costed, outcome-driven, environment: the industrial world of Taylorism that we have been discussing. Some GP practices now display a notice saying that if you have more than one problem you must make two appointments: each appointment lasts only ten minutes. I recently saw a GP who remained standing at her desk, looking down at me throughout the consultation, increasing my sense of time pressure.

Can we afford now to be thinking in terms of personalised relationships at all within NHS general practice, if it is to remain free to all at the point of delivery but is very costly to the nation?

CG: What remains of the NHS was created as the embers of the Second World War died down and there was a spirit of rebuilding—of creating a better, idealistic world. And it belonged to all of us because it was funded through progressive taxation.

This is important because of your comment that it is costly to the nation. It would be even more costly (and unfair in terms of all of our states of health and wealth) if it were not funded through this method. This is why I fought so much during my RCGP Chairmanship. Those socialist ideals (i.e., fair, progressive, value for money), which fitted into our national, post-war British belief system, committed to the greatest good of the greatest number, were under fire.

What was so sad was that many committed MPs in all parties followed their herd leaders, and did not stand by their values. We have all suffered the price: an industrial marketplace drawing on industrial models is replacing our—*yes our*—NHS, of which we were all so proud, and around and within which we felt a sense of collective kinship, as Ballatt and Campling describe.

Dialogue Box 7: Implications of the Consumer Myth

"We are now threatened with the prospect of our only being consumers, able to consume anything from any point in the world and of every culture, but of losing all our originality." (Lévi-Strauss, 1978, p. 20)

MM: Turning to patients now, how would you describe the mental health work carried out by GPs, who are usually the first point of call in community mental health care?

CG: GPs are the main provider of community mental health. We actually provide eighty per cent of this care. There is a wide range of need, from brief, stress-related ill-health (that needs careful diagnosis) to full-blown, severe, chronic mental illness—we cover it all.

The cuts have increased the mental health load. Community care, when it came in in the 1990s, sounded good, but was very seductive because, in reality, it was underfunded, and serious mental health problems were just shunted from the hospitals on to the GP and voluntary organisations, which, because of the new market system, had to make repeated bids for funding (at great cost to themselves). Bidding itself is a very costly process in both human and financial terms. There are now fewer community psychiatric nurses, and mental health provision by other agencies is much thinner than before, and is always changing, due to the perpetual bidding and contracting process, and top-down perverse financial incentives—care incentives barely figure.

MM: I know this too, from supervising frontline therapists who despair at the attitude of their middle-managers trying to meet the targets coming down from on high with decreasing resources, while also trying to keep their careers afloat. The size of waiting lists runs into the hundreds sometimes, and the expected closure rate of their caseloads is barely believable. It bears little relation to the actual nature of mental health problems. I often have to ask my supervisees to repeat the numbers, and the permitted clinical time-spans they report, to make sure I heard correctly.

What would you say are the main stresses that arise for GPs from the large amount of mental health work they carry, and the collaboration with other agencies that it involves, when they are over-stretched themselves? Does psychoanalytic thinking have a contribution to make here, and if so, what has been your experience?

CG: GPs have first to carry grief at the loss of their community role as a kind of sacred healer or father figure, a wise person to whom patients can turn at times of trouble and ill health in their lives. That has pretty much all gone, even if some patients do still put us on a pedestal. More often now, patients are being told by policy-makers, and the media, that GPs are just not doing a good enough job, and many believe it. With this fall from grace comes a loss of that sense of secure attachment, and the all-important containment for the patient, their families, and their community networks—the idea that there is someone there to turn to and count on. In its place, there is a sense that they might be dropped completely, or waiting times might be too long (as now they can be), or that we simply ought to be open longer hours.

In fact, we are already dropping by the wayside ourselves from exhaustion and demoralisation: GPs are leaving the profession in droves. The changes in public perception also add to the kind of distress that is brought through the door: it is less contained, more troubled, because trust has been under fire. *The patient feels all the time that their survival is not safe with us, or the NHS, any more.*

Care of all kinds, health and social, is now provided in a large matrix of care agencies. Wilke, in "Beyond Balint" again, writes about this wider context (your B and C levels) as being something GPs absolutely must now hold in mind, relate to, and work with. Yet, it could be as many as thirty different agencies in a locality (and that is only your B level).

Care is now very fragmented because contracts are always changing with each bidding cycle and there is intense, repetitive, and very wasteful competition for contracts, which does not foster collaboration, even though the work requires it.

Competition is an imperative now, and changes in structures and personnel are too rapid to keep up with. For example, I never know who the IAPT therapist for a patient is, will never meet them. The services are interdependent as far as the patient is concerned, and need to be co-operative, but the way they operate in reality is very fragmented and complex, because it exists in a competitive, not a collaborative, culture.

Social norms have obviously changed too. I think of Elias and the Frankfurt School, writing of how social norms, the manners and conventions of the time, become internalised (Dialogue Box 8).

Dialogue Box 8: Civilisation and its Breakdown

"Elias wrote of the civilising process as an internalisation of various values and forms of social etiquette akin to the super-ego and deriving originally from the court. Originally from Germany, he came to the UK pre-war, to the University of Leicester, and went on to work with Foulkes developing group analysis with a focus on the internalisation of individual and social formations." (Loyal & Quilley, 2004)

In the late 1940s, the NHS values of care and altruism, those post-war socialist ideals, were internalised, but now, since the early 1990s' change to a competitive market culture, it is cost- and efficiency-driven, has a consumerist culture, and a "customer-services-style" complaint system to go with it.

I think people should be able to complain, don't get me wrong, but complaining as a consumer, with a market system in the mind, is quite different to being part of a benevolent NHS kinship network. Complaining as a disappointed patient to someone you still recognise as a true medical professional, with a sense of vocation, is totally different: you both share some idea of what the NHS means, both have a sense of belonging. That changes the mind-set totally, the basic terms of the transaction, the values, are quite different.

The market system puts the doctor on the defensive as they are being judged in terms that come from outside of their professional system, outside of the NHS as we know it. Being a small business, which is what general practice used to be, is not the same as being part of a large business run from elsewhere, by anonymous CCGs and Chief Executive Officers (CEOs) and health business companies. CEOs change jobs frequently, the managerial culture is persecuting and judgemental, and everyone is subject to rapidly changing government policies, affecting how they think, speak, and what they can do. The system is unrecognisable.

I love what I do, more than I can tell you, more than I can explain . . . To be there listening, sharing, thinking deeply about a moment in the life of another human being with them . . . just the two of you. It is *the* most important thing. It *is* sacred, that *is* the right word, but I go home now, and I weep, often. The patients do not see me weep, but I weep. I cannot do the job I love in the way I want to do it any more. So grief is the main stressor. Psychoanalysis has much to say about that.

MM: As a leader within your profession, you have a bird's-eye view of the field as well as a close-up one in clinical practice. Do you think general practice is ever its own "worst enemy"? Have you identified any "social defences", which (while helping the profession to survive twenty-five years of perpetual change within the post-Thatcher market of healthcare) have been detrimental in other ways? If so, can you say anything about what form you think these social defences—or shared "herd"-type behaviours—take?

CG: Maybe I could—but first I want rather to turn this question round, then I want to talk about perverse incentives. I think this is a question, by implication, about what inspires people and what keeps them on task, and what turns them away from their task, undermining their real work.

The Bevin–Beveridge ideals for the early NHS really inspired people; they made doctors want to work for the good of all; they were based on the idea that the health of everyone mattered, including the poorest in our communities (Beveridge, 1942; NHS Act, 1948). The community as a whole was felt to be important. The NHS connected us to each other in a large, kinship network, and GPs were given a vital role within it.

It is quite different now. What is rewarded is activity. We have this industrial model; that is how the system works: by perverse incentives. That is how hospitals bid for, and get paid, in their contracts, for episodes of activity that are costed, counted, and contracted, and ensure their financial viability. They have to earn their keep or go to the wall, go into "special measures".

Dialogue Box 9: Incentive Packages—Envy and Rivalry

"Incentive packages for GPs have been around since 1990 when the first new contract sought to incentivize health promotion by identifying patients at risk. The 2004 contract implemented a fresh approach . . . by micro-managing consultations in selected areas through a complex system of targets . . . These approaches to remunerating work have resulted in unhealthy levels of competitiveness and envy. Most worryingly they have encouraged a negative way of thinking about the job that focuses on onerous tasks rather than the relationship with patients." (Ballatt & Campling, 2011, p. 148)

In the past, GPs obviously were active on behalf of patients, but our job was also felt to be preventive, educative, healing, and if we did it well, and the patient complied, there would actually be *less* activity, which was good because it meant the patient's health improved with a better lifestyle or more knowledge and understanding of their condition, and they saw us less frequently.

Now there are perverse incentives at work, that steer—no, they lead—activity towards ticking boxes, fulfilling contracts, or not overstepping them, ensuring stability of payment for the organisation,

whether a general practice or a hospital. We have to survive financially in our locality, our organisation; we are not free any more to
respond as we feel we should. A perverse incentive constantly pulls
doctors away from their main task. Everything gets out of balance,
distorted, fragmented.

Yet, in spite of the market, in the mind of a GP there has been, and
always will be, space for the idea of being a wounded healer, someone who wants to fix things, repair people who are broken or
damaged in some way, and through doing that sometimes heals themselves, but it always carries the risk of wanting to be all things to all
people: there is the archetypal pull if you like. That takes us off task,
because we cannot be that person, we are only human, and do not
have that godlike power. When the archetypal myth gets hold of us,
we just work harder and harder and harder, all hours, get sick and
depressed, do a less good job, because we can never be that mythic
figure that took us into the profession in the first place.

That we live in a tick-box market-world encourages unhealthy
(mechanical and omnipotent) defences, that eat up our time in mindless ways. As I said earlier, there are over thirty NHS regulators we
have to answer to, report back to, at present—all of whom have soft-
ware packages that are part of our daily working lives. Can you imagine that? People have even lost track of how many there are, and it is
always changing. Every piece of activity is measured, weighed, and
costed, compared with some indicator. There is no coherence what-
soever. You can see how easy it is to get lost, waylaid, or exhausted,
on things far removed from our first task, the job I said I love so much:
seeing patients, and caring for them in the best possible way.

Dialogue Box 10 " Something Is Profoundly Wrong"

"Something is profoundly wrong with the way we live today. For
thirty years we have made a virtue out of the pursuit of material self-
interest: indeed, this very pursuit now constitutes whatever remains
of our sense of collective purpose. We know what things cost but
have no idea what they are worth." (Judt, 2010) (See also Gerada,
2014)

MM: Clare, I want to change key now, to something more positive: can
you say something briefly about the best of general practice today?

CG: Well, there are many ways to answer this question—and other people have done so—but I am not going to be academic or technical about it. It is simple really: I love my profession and I love my job. As do most, if not all, of my colleagues.

General practice at its best is about love and care, in addition to clinical competence, and good time management: the love we have for one another, and the way we care for our community, and each other in our profession. But it is all under fire, that is why people are leaving, and recruitment is low.

MM: You have supported the "intelligent kindness" and "global compassion" agendas in mental health (Ballatt & Campling, 2011; Pietroni, 2015). Are these recent positive agendas the beginning of a genuine rebalancing of the values that drive policy and practice in health and social care, here and worldwide? Or are there risks here, if they, too, become used as political spin, or institutionalised?

CG: Well, there is a risk. They must not be institutionalised, must not be used as spin. People have projected into Corbyn their hopes for the future, and he has been attacked by a right-wing press, mercilessly. We deserve better. We must protect the good, identify the good, fight for the good, because it is under attack from all sides at present.

Everyone has their corruption point, and all the more so when morale is so low, and we now spend most of our time doing work which is not related to our patients in any tangible way, much of it on the computer being regulated, and our output measured against various criteria.

How can you measure sustaining clinical relationships? How can they be measured and counted? How can we protect the sacred space between doctor and patient when every aspect of it is being fragmented and fed into a computer?

Yesterday, I sat down with an Iraqi refugee and her child, and I asked her where she had come from, and why she had come to see me. I was there for half an hour, and it should have been longer. She told me her extraordinary story. How can we measure or cost that encounter, what contract can it fit into, even if we know it relates directly to health, and to mental health, because the research is clear? Compassion and kindness should never be the subject of political spin. They cannot be measured. No tick-box will show those outcomes.

As David Himmelstein, the founder of Health Maintenance Organisation, said: healthcare is like blood. It is too intimate, too precious, and too easily corruptible to be left to the market. That idea is so important—I have it on my Apple watch so I never forget it, it is like a mantra, I keep repeating it.

CHAPTER TWELVE

General practice, mental health, and stress. Part 2: organisational model and commentary on the postmodern context

Marilyn Miller

And we are here as on a darkling plain
Swept with confused alarms of struggle and flight,
Where ignorant armies clash by night

(Dover Beach [1867] in Dwight Culler, 1961)

Preamble

This chapter is divided into two parts. First, general practice takes place within an organisational context that needs to be taken into account. The simple ABC organisational model, referred to in the dialogue, is here described in more detail, identifying three levels of professional activity. These levels both differentiate and link areas of activity and their associated work roles. The fluent integration of the political with research and practice in Dr Gerada's answers almost obscures the way she moves through the hierarchical levels from front-line clinical practice, right up to a top-level, national, leadership role, and back again. The ABC model here seeks to make the organisational complexity underpinning her fluency more explicit.

The second part provides a commentary on the dialogue using psychoanalytic concepts, particularly containment, which are essential to mental health work, and discusses the implications of its absence in the "new NHS" conditions, for patient and GP alike.

The argument as a whole is then placed within the socio-historical context of "postmodernity", taken here to mean a superficial culture, driven by market principles, and littered confusingly with archaic throwbacks, odd juxtapositions, and linguistic gimmicks.

Part I: The ABC of organisational life— a spatial model to hold in mind

The ABC model differentiates three levels of professional activity in much the same way as thinking about families requires separating the generations in one's mind, while being fully aware of how they link and interact. The model works at the level of an ideogram: loosely, offering a tool for navigating what can often seem like organisational "fog" in the NHS. It is simple, but designed to illuminate highly complex processes.

The model was originally developed as a response to the challenges of being a senior manager, across mental health services provided by two highly bureaucratised but interacting large organisations and their surrounding local agencies (a teaching hospital, St Bartholomew's, and social services department, the City of London, along with other community agencies). The model was inspired by a wish to simplify Eliot Jaques' stratified systems theory, and his detailed work on timespans of discretion, decision-making, and individual capacity in relation to hierarchy, in order to make it more useable on an everyday basis (Miller, 1975).

Jaques' model emphasised time; the ABC model emphasises space, simply identifying the different spaces in which professional activity takes place. Space here, because defined ideogrammatically, is considered to be both mental and geographical, an internal metaphor and an operational reality (thus, A: same room; B: locality-based; C: national in scope). In current working environments, as Dr Gerada describes, mental space too often seems in short supply, and these settings operate under a great deal of pressure.

The more for less efficiency aims of the NHS market environment have seen a vast range of bureaucratic, computerised systems established at each of the B and C levels. Dr Gerada refers to over thirty regulatory bodies but the total number and their individual purposes are hard to grasp and understand, especially in the NHS hotbed of perpetual change. For example, even the NHS's own organisational website had recently not managed to change the names of Monitor and the four other organisations with which it had recently merged to make up the new organisation: NHS Improvement. Officially, this change occurred almost a month ago at the time of writing, but the computerised information systems designed to support professional operations had not caught up. If one combines this relatively small reality with the bigger one—that the aims and real-life tasks of these now morphed organisations had themselves not yet been adequately known or understood (and will undoubtedly change again shortly)—the result is a confusing context where the parts cannot be differentiated or appropriately related within the whole. A sense of perspective that allows part and whole to be held in mind is therefore lost.

Rapid policy change thus creates a rapidly moving "virtual world". Confusing differentiations and mergers create a perverse environmental context, at B and C levels, akin to the incestuous family where appropriate generational roles and behaviours have been lost, and the time-based developmental needs of different life stages have been bypassed. "Naming the parts" is sometimes impossible in such hotbeds of policy change, as the above example shows. The result can be disorientation, distress, and mindlessness, which are wholly dysfunctional in health care.

The insistent computerised demands of these changing systems of regulation now occupy the precious interstices of everyday professional space. That space was previously available for reflection, and for digesting and thinking through the emotional impact of often distressing work, as well as for ordinary, productive collegiate interaction. Using the interstices of work in this way is not time-wasting or inefficient, as the Taylorist industrial models imply; on the contrary, it helps clarify thinking, and aids mindfulness. These previously spontaneous marginal activities offered an essential space for self-containment, allowing a self-regulating internal and interpersonal process to happen quite naturally. Without that free space on the "edges" and "in-betweens" of work, distressing, intimate healthcare activities remain undigested and become "crammed" internally. The additional demands of repetitive data entry activity (for the "bureau" of C and B level control and command systems) leave the inner need for self-containment and self-regulation unmet: the consequence is that ordinary human needs are rendered nugatory.

That data must be collected, analysed, and appropriately used for improving services and making best use of scarce resources is not in doubt, but healthcare is not a factory operation. It deals with human beings and their physical and mental needs, sometimes of an extreme kind around birth and death, or trauma, or pain and chronic illness, or disability. It is often distressing and intimate and evokes deeply personal responses (Menzies Lyth, 1988a,b[1959a,b]). The end result of squeezing out thinking time and excessively duplicating data collection for Levels C and B is a failure to allow sufficient fallow time at level A for recovery and regeneration. Mindless activity of the counting and collecting kind, as described by Menzies Lyth, can then become an end in itself, rather than serving, as it should, the primary tasks of healthcare and the necessary subsidiary tasks of caring for staff (Figure 12.1).

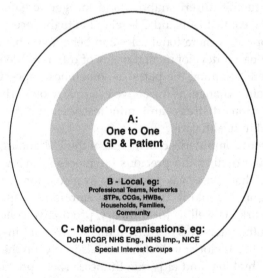

A:
One to One
GP & Patient

B - Local, eg:
Professional Teams, Networks
STPs, CCGs, HWBs,
Households, Families,
Community

C - National Organisations, eg:
DoH, RCGP, NHS Eng., NHS Imp., NICE
Special Interest Groups

The ABC of Organisational Life:
'Top Down & Bottom Up'

(Individual, Small Group and Large
Group Phenomena)

Figure 12.1.   The ABC of organisational life—a spatial model to hold in mind.

The ABC model offers a simple map for remaining in touch with this top-down working reality for front-line general practice: there are co-existing policy and practice "shapers" at the B and C levels, operating in parallel and simultaneously. These "shaping" organisations also tend to function as independent "silos", fermenting their own ideas in their own different time frames, making joined-up thinking very difficult for the practitioner to achieve. This fragmentation leaves the GP (and other front-line workers) bearing the strain of the duplications and contradictions that result, and promotes deadening routines rather than refined clinical thought.

At a recent NHS Improvement conference for Trust and Foundation Trust governors, the radically new models of organisation proposed in the NHS Five Year Forward View (NHS, 2014) were shown to include new forms of vertical and horizontal integration, which were questioned by Trust governors because they were "bringing back" the principle of *collaboration*. The governors pointed out to the NHS representative that, in practice (at the A and B levels), an actual court case had not long before resulted when inter-agency providers were deemed to be promoting *collaboration* and ignoring the then paramount policy imperative of market *competition*. The NHS manager responded by shrugging, when confronted with this now confusing top-down anomaly between the principles of competition and collaboration, saying it would "all be worked out at ground level" (A and B levels) and that the policy-makers (C Level) would listen and respond positively to innovations they deemed to be effective in practice. These innovative models would then become "standard bearers for the future". Not knowing if certain forms of collaborative practice will be met by a court case or by applause is an example of the "suck it and see", top-down policy contradictions that sap morale and erode motivation at Level A, where the emotional impact of the work itself and the thoughtful collaborations it requires are a real, daily experience.

Policy implementation takes time to be established, to be "threaded through", so when policy change from Level C is top-down and rapid, it disrupts and can foreclose slower-moving implementation processes at Levels B and A. For example, when Primary Care Trusts (PCTs) were required to give way to Clinical Commissioning Groups (CCGs), C level national policy change superseded earlier developments at the local B level, which were just beginning to mature. At times, those now established CCGs (at the B level) change existing contracts with established front-line A and B level providers, disturbing much-needed continuity of care and delicate inter-agency collaboration. However, the results of contract change still have to be worked with, and new collaborations have to be established, creating recurring waves of stress and disorientation to all concerned. GPs and their practices, as Dr Gerada describes, are often struggling to survive in this harsh new NHS, with its financially driven policy changes, which, because they are not co-ordinated, can collide messily within and between all three A, B, and C systems.

These collision processes between the different levels and paces of policy implementation are reminiscent of Bion's description, in his paper on psychotic thought processes, of "agglomeration" or "cruel linking" (1959). Rapid and incessant policy change with annual efficiency savings, changing targets, and perverse financial incentives, each implemented through computerised systems, creates a complex, multi-level, organisational environment that is too often inimical to thought, and reflects the absence of any overarching policy change thinker or thought process. In short, it can and does feel crazy much of the time.

Professional roles within the ABC system

At each of the three organisational levels, the GP's different professional "selves" can be activated as they fill different roles: the personal and professional self at Level A, the local team-playing and networking self at Level B, and the national, political self at Level C.

Personal choices about the alternative group roles of member, follower, and leader are ideally to be made in the "small group" life of Level B, and the "large group" life of Level C. However, as Dr Gerada's answers suggest, such choices these days have to be more expedient, influenced as they are not only by the survival needs of the individual but also by those of their professional group or tribe: general practice. The rate of exit from general practice and serious difficulties with recruitment, which are reflected in the GP Forward View proposals, brought out only in April 2016, seek to respond to a crisis in general practice. A nationwide counselling service has since been provided to assist.the retention of GPs, led by Dr Gerada's Hurley Group. Urgent re-financing and new recruitment policies now come with this new staff support provision in a fairly desperate attempt to stem the flight, which Dr Gerada attributes to fear that is now "the emotional driver at all organisational levels: individually in the consulting room, in the professional grapevines, in local groups and networks, or in the dreams and nightmares of policy-makers as they introduce yet another fanfared change of structure and language".

Part II: Commentary on the dialogue with Dr Gerada

Continuity of care

Dr Gerada identifies continuity of care as the defining feature of general practice. She explains how it permits GPs to work in a relationship with their patients over time, and to show depth and detailed understanding of body and mind, and of family and social networks across generations: all of this within what is usually a ten-minute consultation.

Such continuity ensures that a particular quality of thought is developed within the brief time frame available, and can be sustained between GP and patient: a *safe* time–space that fosters communication and the more intuitive aspects of a bio-psycho-social assessment.

Continuity of care, thus, allows GPs to perform at their highest levels of competence, using their experience, skills, and knowledge to the full. They can build a life-history narrative that evolves over time, in which each episode of GP contact, and of ill health, can more easily be understood. While a "fresh eye" from a colleague can often be useful, continuity is usually to the greatest advantage of the patient as it fosters the linking of body and mind in diagnosis.

In psychoanalytic treatment, continuity is a given, albeit around a quite different clinical task: one that is focused on the mind and does not require the expert scanning of the body and a swift and appropriate body–mind response. Nevertheless, like the Balints (Balint, 1955), we can assume that the core knowledge about how body and mind interact, and some of the diagnostic realities then implicated, also apply to general practice. Sanders (1984) has explained this process in detail in his book, *A Matter of Interest: Clinical Notes of a Psycho-analyst in General Practice*, where he uses the term "protomental" (drawing on Bion and Meltzer) to convey the depth and complexity of the body–mind presentation with which GPs are daily faced.

Continuity of care, one can therefore say, protects the conditions needed for containment of pre/unconscious communication between two people and fosters the emergence of deeper thinking about body–mind interactions. "Thinking together" productively is also more likely to occur, adding a developmental, dynamic opportunity for both doctor and patient—as, for example, in Dr Gerada's example of the mother fearing for the safety of her child after an earlier child's death. In contrast, a more static, scientific model, based entirely on "expert and patient", tends to increase investigations (and, hence, costs), leaving the more subtle zones of body–mind expression unexamined.

The container–contained relationship and the NHS

Containment is also central, and goes hand in hand with continuity of care. As Dr Gerada explains, the NHS, as an organisation, once acted as a shared container for our communal fear of death. GPs are the defining "hubs" of clinical activity within the large and highly complex NHS system: they assess on first contact, sustain over years, refer to secondary care where necessary, and follow-up on discharge. They respond to birth, illness, and life changes, and to death; to body and to mind.

Dr Gerada reminds us of how, before the market system was introduced, we put our faith and trust in the NHS as a national institution based on humanitarian values, which we invested with pride and affection, and from which we derived a communal sense of safety. The "new NHS" has been transformed into a more impersonal, commercial organisation, run on industrial lines. The NHS market and its private finance initiative (PFI) has also been used to attract global business partners, particularly from the USA (Pollitt & Bouckaert, 2004). As Illiffe (2008) describes, this industrialised commercial model means that the NHS is no longer easily able to fulfil its containing function.

As a consequence, we, as individuals, are now more likely to be left with a sense of being alone with our mental and bodily changes and fears. This sense of aloneness is increased with the frequent crises now besetting the NHS, such as the junior doctors' first ever strike to affect emergency services (April 2016). This loss of background containment, with its accompanying sense of insecurity and discontinuity in the wider NHS, increases the internal level of ordinary survival fear that each of us has not had to carry, and which, from time to time, we might embody in symptoms. We may take this primitive fear as an "illness" to our GPs, in undifferentiated "protomental" or psychosomatic form, as Sanders (1984) describes. Reading the body–mind relationship, therefore, as Dr Gerada did in the example of the mother and daughter presentation, is key to the rapid assessment every GP must make. Throughout, however, GPs must also be ready to identify potentially significant physical or mental illness, and react or refer accordingly. It is a tall order in the best of conditions . . .

In the days of Balint, the dynamic transference and countertransference of the doctor–patient relationship was itself seen as the containing vessel for resolving, and working through, the range of "protomental" anxieties that we express in complex ways, and for differentiating them from more significant organic illness. Now, however, the GP-patient relationship is burdened by many additional layers of organisational complexity, as Dr Gerada carefully points out (Wilke et al., 2000).

The loss of this background containing function by the NHS has been caused in part by the rapid and disorientating policy and structural changes between 1990 and 2015, since the introduction, under Margaret Thatcher, of the internal market. The market itself has had more impact, due to the level of technological change. The ebb and flow of pessimism and optimism, which accompanies Dr Gerada's answers, is tangible: it reflects the ebb and flow of the continuity of her lifelong professional commitment, and her struggle with the de-skilling realities that now abound. Not only does she demonstrate self-sustainment at work, within this complexity, she also shares with us a movement back and forth along the paranoid schizoid—depressive continuum: her self-containment is sure, but turbulent, and under fire (Bion, 1963).

Things not people: paranoid anxiety, fragmentation, reification

The NHS, as originally conceived, developed into a culturally unifying, humanitarian force, drawing on labour from all over the world; some would say it was one of the more successful stories of our multi-cultural society. It was not, however, without its faults; our national class structures, and associated privileges and condescensions were also displayed, along with undue institutional tolerance of elitist practices.

These class-based issues (military style ward rounds, consultants AWOL during the cricket season, tolerance of the excesses of deferential and arrogant behaviour, silence on doctor and nurse addictions, out-patients given all the same appointment time and expected to wait) were common in the period between 1948 and 1990, and they should not be forgotten.

The NHS bonds, at the same time, were undoubtedly life sustaining for staff and patients, and profoundly relational. That network has given way, over the past twenty-five years, to impersonal business units with complex, and at times hard to decipher, infrastructures. Trusts and Foundation Trusts, Clinical Commissioning Groups, Sustainability and Transformation Plans, and so forth, form part of a competitive internal market, enshrined in law and regulated by national bodies working within the austerity constraints of HM Treasury. Mysterious acronyms abound.

The old NHS kinship systems, with their innate familiarity, taken-for-granted flaws and connectedness, and "benefit of the doubt" form of trust, do still survive, and even thrive in some areas, but have too often been eroded, or simply broken up. In place of kinship, the current competitive working conditions of the NHS, together with their constant subjection to inspection checks, tend to generate fear and suspicion, and, therefore, loneliness.

In these competitive, business-style conditions, the potential for joined-up thinking from (or about) the over thirty regulators that oversee NHS trusts and general practice is virtually nil. Instead, these powerfully fragmenting and quite impersonal forces, coming in from above and outside, foreground abstract numerical data, "traffic light" quality ratings, and cost-effectiveness. This form of regulation is too often disconnected from its human implications, and deeply undermines any sense of an available NHS safety net. It adds an alien quality, a less than humanitarian force, to the increased inner fears about life and death that patients and GPs now have to carry in their clinical encounters.

A sense of perspective, and a capacity for continuing, deeper levels of thought is hard for any practitioner to sustain in these circumstances. Fragmentation and unhealthy splitting can easily result, as the survival fear that GPs widely report becomes paramount. Thus, the vicious circles associated with these primitive mental processes— a state of mind characterised by fear, shame, and the need to blame— can take over: containment has then been lost.

These are the features of reification—or "part object/thing-thinking"—where the focus is on parts, on things, on isolated functions, rather than whole living persons. These are the conditions revealed by Lord Francis's *Report of the Mid Staffordshire NHS Foundation Trust Public Inquiry* (2013), in which human beings and their healthcare problems can be turned in the mind into a horde of "things that persecute", or, to use Bion's terms, "the furniture of dreams" in a mental universe of "bizarre objects" (1967). The Francis Report provides a frightening case study of where this primitive state of mind can lead, and deserves careful reading.

Dr Gerada's reference to the term "aliquots of health care" is a clear example of this process of "thing-thinking". The phrase generates an oddly estranging effect: "aliquot" means a part of a greater whole—a part object, in fact—so human beings are redefined as small, composite samples of a health budget working in practice. The somewhat puzzling cryptic language used here, in the national discourse of regulating cost effectiveness, might be more at home in a Beckett play (that presents and exploits estrangement) than in a general practice that runs on the best of humanitarian endeavour, even if far from perfect.

It is not that hard to see how, in this highly competitive financial environment, the NHS has been transformed into a system in which patients—human beings—are reduced to health-care cost-samples and (dehumanised now further by language) subjected to the kind of neglect and ill-treatment described in the Francis Report: "The Trust prioritised its finances and its Foundation Trust application over its quality of care and failed to put its patients first" (Francis, 2013, p. 15); also, "Monitor focused on finance and corporate governance as opposed to patient safety and quality" (Francis, 2013, p. 15). Cost priorities have replaced human ones, and human beings are lost in this somewhat dysfunctional large system, whose core values and daily practices have changed beyond recognition. Paranoid anxiety is such that "things" can seem both worse than they are, and better than they are, at one and the same time, and very confusingly.

The use of metaphor as a "transitional" container

So, where can containment be found?

Dr Gerada frequently finds containment—and offers it to us—in metaphor, sometimes inspirationally, and usually provocatively, illuminating our thoughts.

There is an emerging consensus that metaphor, which links two unfamiliar ideas that nevertheless share some common properties, is often used to grasp and hold elusive experiences (Enckell, 2002; Lakoff & Johnson, 1980, 1999; Sharpe, 1940). There is also a consensus that, while our use of metaphor can open up understanding, it can also do the opposite—foreclosing thought. Metaphor can act as a useful, pictorial, verbal container for unfamiliar experiences that we are reaching to describe and understand, using categories and terms that are familiar to us. Metaphors can graphically hold and "name the parts" for us—bits of semi-digested or simplified experience, and "just developing ideas"—while showing some appreciation of the complexity of "the whole", to which these parts belong. They offer graphic expression that can act as a temporary stepping-stone to deeper understanding and articulation.

The nature of the metaphor, however, also matters. Dr Gerada uses many strong metaphors: politicians as spoilt children wanting their own way or as dogs peeing on lamp-posts; GPs as battered wives and children, naughty children, helpless abused orphans, scapegoats like social workers; general practice as a factory production line, or veering between black cab and Uber cabs in a taxi-rank model of practice; and "Kwikfit" IAPT psychotherapy. The NHS is described as an old, stately home now stripped of windows, doors, and cornerstones, or a two-tier flight system where only the first-class passengers are carried, and others left on the tarmac.

The movement in Dr Gerada's argument—from more human, bodily, and familiar metaphors, towards mechanical and industrial ones—is telling (hence my dialogue boxes dropped in as nudging notations, and now these accompanying arguments about confusions of purpose and task generated by a dehumanising process at work). Her extensive use of metaphor is itself, one can argue, a means of surviving, holding on to, and communicating an intense humanity in "word pictures", when the NHS, and general practice within it, have become so dehumanised and "strange", and, at times, so threatened and threatening. This is the profession that she grew up to *love*, following in her father's footsteps, and still loves, and pours love into daily, but must now spend much of her life fighting to protect, while many other GPs can barely survive. Her graphic use of metaphor is able to contain some fairly disturbing ideas, while, at the same time, it provides positive stepping-stones for thought, and, just as importantly, wider communication, reaching people emotionally, making them think, in conditions that militate against both thought and communication.

The metaphors make creative use, in psychoanalytic terms, of primary and secondary process, and offer a breathing space for what Bion described as "alpha function" to take place, so that the "thing-thinking/beta elements" can be transformed. Here, the creative thought of one individual in a leadership role reaches out more easily across the profession; the internal recovery of the large group (the profession of general practice), as well as the individual, is, therefore, offered a helping hand.

These vivid metaphors are made to work hard at containment, offering a life raft for all to cling to, when thought (and humanity itself) is under fire, at the same time as making it possible sometimes to say the unsayable. After all, what Dr Gerada calls the delicate "eco-system" of our NHS is at risk, if it is not already, like the effects of climate change, too late.

The limits of human perception in our postmodern world

Dialogue Box 11 : Post-modernism and the evolution of perception

"I am proposing the notion that we are in the presence of something like a mutation ... My implication is that we ourselves, the human subjects who happen to inhabit this new space, have not kept pace with evolution; there has been a mutation in the object unaccompanied as yet by any equivalent mutation in the subject. We do not possess the perceptual equipment to match this new hyperspace ... in part because our perceptual habits were formed in that older kind of space ... (we need to) grow new organs, to expand our sensorium and our body to some new, yet unimaginable, perhaps ultimately impossible, dimensions." (Jameson, 1991, pp. 38–39)

"Postmodernity: a superficial culture, driven by market principles, and littered confusingly with archaic throwbacks, odd juxtapositions, and linguistic gimmicks." (Miller, see page 214, current volume)

Here, I want to locate the above discussion in a wider context by juxtaposing Jameson's lucid, 1991 analysis of our postmodern, Western culture, with Dr Gerada's vivid, 2016 descriptions of everyday general practice. The dates span the key developmental period of the new NHS and its internal market.

Jameson refers to a process of critical change, a "mutation", which he links with what he calls elsewhere the "cultural logic of late capitalism", an ideology which he sees permeating all aspects of our culture. The NHS policy changes, beginning in 1990 with the Griffiths' Report, introduced a supermarket model into healthcare—after Roy Griffiths' Sainsbury connection. What we used to think of as "our NHS", with its shared sense of a safety net and of kinship networks that drew us together, seems quietly over this period to have developed into a fear-laden, sometimes lethal organisation, which constantly changes "the names of its parts" and the way they connect in practice, in confusing ways.

Every parent knows how important the developmental stage of naming body parts is—nose, mouth, ear, finger, toe, and so forth—in enabling their infant to become orientated, and to have a developing sense of their enduring but bounded existence with familiar and reassuring daily rhythms and structures, and eventually to communicate to others using a shared language. This primary experience allows us to live and work from "within our own skin" and to "have a mind of our own" with which we can think.

When national policy changes terminology so frequently that it requires the regular publication of new glossaries of the terms in use, and long lists of acronyms that also change and are now often used in lieu of words, it is easy to see how professionals, however strong their primary foundation, can be thrust back into states of infant-like disorientation and helplessness. This state is not just a feeling or a sensation. As Dr Gerada describes, and the Francis Report and junior doctors' strike bear out, there is indeed a loss of control, in which GPs too often find themselves in a working environment where new structures and language are routinely imposed. GPs are, thus, along with others, deskilled and estranged from the shared values and language of their professional family and the familiar daily rhythms that sustain their working patterns.

As one whole system of policy change is almost mastered, and a new language learnt, so a new policy change repeats the disorientating process, starting again with naming (and coding with acronyms) new parts, dividing and ruling, insiders who are in the know from outsiders who are not. These ever-emerging parts of the NHS, whether in general practice or among the mental health services, must then again be named and reconfigured into a new whole, within the mind of each practitioner. Language can, therefore, no longer be relied on, is never a constant; structures of thought and feeling must be frequently reconfigured; working continuities are disrupted—at great cost to both the individual and the wider system. It is more than a little "mad-making".

It is hardly surprising, then, that a recent survey found 74.7% of West Midlands GPs believed their workload to be "unmanageable", leading local medical committees to hold emergency meetings to demand urgent action to reduce their burdens, and the BMA's GP Executive Committee to declare a state of emergency in general practice (McCarron, 2015).

Jameson proposes that our Western, "hi-tech" culture is confusing (the NHS and its frequent policy changes is but one example), because the speed and nature of change has outstripped our human capacity for adaptation. He describes how a loss of perspective follows, because human perception has been unable to keep up with the depersonalising effects of this rapid-change, "push-button", "instant everything", "cash-driven", materialistic world. The "must have it now" mental states that are developmentally normal for early infancy then infect and undermine the minds and working cultures of professional adults, removing the sustaining effects of continuities of all kinds, and creating a working environment which feels insecure, foreign, and uncomfortable much of the time.

Jameson's description of the prevailing culture resonates with Klein's description (1933) of how, in the absence of perceptual integration, and the presence of developmentally "natural" omnipotent thinking, characteristic of the first three to six months of life, disorientating part-object relationships prevail. Whole-object, three-dimensional thinking, with a sense of perspective, has not yet been established. It is as if, in reaching forward to survive in this alienating, new NHS-market world, we are also obliged to reach backwards to our earliest experience, and can easily get lost in the process, in a kind of "back to the future" effect.

Computerisation has accelerated and complicated this "mutation in the [e.g., NHS object]" that Jameson describes, not least because of the chaotically multiplied, "top-down", regulatory uses to which it has been put (driven by the values of the market culture). Local and national regulatory data systems are too rarely "in sync". Duplications and cross-purposes therefore abound, and tend to create a set of unremitting, daily, somewhat deadening behavioural norms and mind-sets, whose demoralising force is most acutely experienced by GPs because they are at the hub of the massive NHS system and themselves link the parts of that system to the whole.

Audit: listening to the system?

Continuing Jameson's theme of perception, the regulatory, computerised, audit processes of the NHS can often seem alien from the root meaning: *audire* (Latin: "to hear"). Audit, as practised, more often provides another example of how an opportunity for listening in depth, followed by productive thought, has instead become a superficial, deadening, "tick-box" activity.

As I noted earlier, listening to flows of clinical activity, and using the information and understanding gained to steer resources where they are most needed, is important. The clinical significance of data, however, is too often trumped by cost significance, not least because, as the Francis Report found, the two functions of cost and clinical care have been organisationally separated, both nationally at regulator level (C level), and locally (B level).

Like all other parts of the NHS, general practice is rigorously audited. We have heard how over thirty "regulators" require regular information, and that no one body has an adequate overview—no one knows how many there are or what exact purpose all serve. Duplications and systematic, bureaucratic inertia are, therefore, rife. Daily data entry proliferates, and easily becomes an excessively time-consuming activity, especially with frequent changes of priority, terminology, and data system. GPs and other NHS practitioners, including IAPT psychotherapists, are required (in seemingly robotic fashion) to enter such data, whether or not it will be sufficiently listened to, or its purpose properly known and fed back to them. As Dr Gerada has described from the "real-life" NHS Listening Events, the cumulative effect of these estranging processes is a generalised fear of annihilation.

There are very serious implications here for the health and welfare of highly trained GPs, and the sustainability of good professional practice—not least for the use and misuse of precious resources, and perhaps even for the survival of the NHS itself.

A tipping point within an NHS "running on love"?

It is widely reported by senior NHS managers that, as a result of the conditions described above, an organisational breakdown of the NHS is possible, or even likely. For example, the British Medical Association has declared a crisis in general practice created by people leaving the profession, difficulties in recruitment, and demoralisation and stress caused by excessive workload and a "pointless" box-ticking culture (McCarron, 2015). If such reports are taken seriously, the seemingly innocent, silent activity of fragmented, parallel, mass audits will have played no small part in creating the anti-life, mechanised conditions where the breakdown of individual human beings and their surrounding large system is more likely to happen. Frequent policy change, using language that is not only elusive, but also regularly erased before it has been fully established, adds to the current fragility of the NHS; so, also, does the kind of structural change marked out by the trail leading from GP fund-holding, Primary Care Trusts, Clinical Commissioning Groups, and various other forms of GP federation.

Tipping points are often characterised by a "regression" to herd behaviour (safety in numbers), the erosion and loss of higher functions of thought (the takeover of simple slogans and political spin), and primal behaviours, where survival strategies take over from communication.

It is, for the most part, a rather bleak picture of a professional environment that is sometimes riskily out of control, even if pockets of normality and some new breakthroughs still exist.

Yet, there is also much to be inspired by in Dr Gerada's account. She repeatedly resuscitates professional self-esteem, and asserts the value of real observation and listening, of properly processing experience, of using psychoanalytic concepts such as projective identification and containment in an integrated way with research evidence and other conceptual frameworks. She insists on going on with deep thinking and feeling, rather than shrink from it, even though she weeps as a result in private. On this foundation of integrated thought, resilience can be generated, and then again regenerated. From the start, her perspectives are multi-level: clinical, local, and national. We witness her actively seeking to protect, and heal, the broken spirit and lost values of the "old" NHS, by strong appeals to, and expressions of, love and care, for individual patients, for general practice, for her profession, and for the values of the old NHS. She also makes clear that protecting and caring for oneself as a practitioner is fundamental, and essential to good practice.

From her account, general practice, one could say, in truth, is still vocational, running on love as much as, if not more than, it runs on money: without love it could not survive in today's conditions. Yet, love is not a recordable or quantifiable resource any more than it is amenable to regulation.

There is here a life-affirming determination to hold on to, protect, and assert "the good object" of general practice as the hub of the NHS, and to resist the faceless, competition-driven forces of a creeping global market and silent privatisation, of ceaseless policy and language change, of excessive regulation, and of perverse incentives. As she says, "We must protect the good, identify the good, fight for the good, because it is under fire from all sides."

Conclusion

Dr Gerada was, until 2013, the elected leader of forty thousand GPs, with the authority to speak for them all. Her successors are making the same warnings as she does, and describing the same conditions.

In her dialogue with me, she shows us a chaotic battle, between the life and death instincts, that is being played out at the general practice hub of our "new NHS". The cost-led internal market, with its industrial contracting and regulatory systems, is now part of a wider global market of healthcare, often driven by international business interests and financial imperatives. Competition is obligatory, and perverse incentives abound. Only the strongest individuals and organisations can survive in a culture that is often inimical to fellow-feeling, to a sense of kinship.

This state of affairs was foretold by Jameson (1991), writing on our postmodern world, as the inevitable "cultural logic of late capitalism". And, as long ago as 1978, Lévi-Strauss warned that, in an "over-communicating" culture, we could be reduced to mere consumers, losing our sense of perspective and our unique human capacity for original thought. Now Dr Gerada and her successors are warning us—and recent surveys have also revealed (NHS, 2014)—that the new

NHS business culture is tearing apart GPs and other workers within it. Without the loving commitment of these workers, there is a real question whether general practice could survive.

CHAPTER THIRTEEN

Concluding remarks

Alison Vaspe

This book set out with Freud's vision of publicly funded treatment for the minds of all who needed it, both rich and poor. Thirty years after his speech, in the country to which he turned as a refugee, the NHS was founded, not just for medical treatment, but also in order to provide just such a service for psychological problems—sadly, too late for Freud to witness it.

Mental health services are now part of our expectation as a society that we have a place in which patients can be cared for and treatment provided, without charge, in the hope that they can be made well enough to return to their lives, with their ordinary forms of support, and sometimes with continuing forms of specialised help. The implicit promise of these services is that another mind is prepared to bear what the patient's cannot. As Joanne Stubley writes, simply and movingly, for refugees this psychological and emotional containment "is something that I feel is part of providing a home—hopefully a temporary one—for what cannot yet be borne". Those who suffer in their minds require this form of asylum, as a refuge from mental pain that can feel unendurable and is often disabling.

Mental health workers aim to relieve the suffering of their patients and to help them to develop better ways of relating, to themselves and to others. The raw states of mind involved in, for example, depressive breakdown, where the patient is subject to terrible, unreasoning guilt, or the self-hatred and disgust of those who harm themselves, involve unconscious beliefs, phantasies, and perceptions, often with dangerous consequences for the sufferer or for those around them. In the Introduction, I suggested that the unconscious mind, like the wild tiger, may be both dangerous and elusive, but it is also a sign of inner life. When we are mentally well, it is the source of our potential for love and creativity. When we are not, it can distort what is good in the life around us, including the love of those who try to care.

These staff are faced on a daily basis with the task of caring for psychological suffering, which may present as destructive or hopeless. As Marilyn Miller described in Chapter One, not all patients can be helped in ways that transform their experience for the better. This is painful to accept, but it is essential that we do so, if patients are not to be seen by those charged with their care as successes or failures. In order to find this acceptance, staff members have to find ways of managing their own difficult and disturbing feelings in response to their patients, and these include frustration and disappointment. As Bell wrote, in a valuable discussion of "Mental illness and its treatment today" (2013), we need to spare these staff the strain of supporting a social "myth" that all patients "can and must recover—and in short order . . . much of the care of the mentally ill centres upon damage limitation and rehabilitation, but not on cure" (Bell, 2013).

The *Five Year Forward View for Mental Health*, from the Independent Mental Health Taskforce to the NHS in England (2016), makes important points about the needs of mental health staff, including the "need to be treated with compassion":

> The care they receive impacts on the care they are able to deliver. Ten million working days are lost each year to sickness absence in the NHS. Some 43 per cent of mental health staff cite work related stress as the cause . . . Findings from the British Psychological Society and New Savoy staff wellbeing survey for 2015 show that around half of psychological professionals surveyed report depression. Seventy per cent say they are finding their job stressful. Yet the quality of the NHS occupational health service is inconsistent and, in some cases, inadequate, according to the NHS Health and Wellbeing Review. (p. 45)

And:

> Protecting the mental health of the workforce is also vital. NHS England has committed to helping staff make choices to improve their own health, and mental health is a key part of that. This should apply across the NHS . . . Every NHS trust should become an "enabling" environment, as recommended in the Francis Report, so people want to work there. Trusts should monitor the mental health of their staff and provide effective occupational health services. (p. 47)

However, this book shows that attention has to be paid to the staff, not just outside the workplace, but also within it. As Cooper and Lousada (2005) remind us, "For mental health clinicians the work, if done well, disturbs the practitioner" (p. 113). Like the contributors to this book, they note the unconscious wish in us all to turn away from psychological experiences that are difficult and unsettling:

> It is a telling aspect of contemporary organizational practice that so many are sent home, or excuse themselves from work with stress, as if being at home will address what is stressful and anxiety-provoking about the task and the system in which anxiety is purportedly contained. (Cooper & Lousada, 2005, p. 113)

This is the context in which the psychoanalytic focus on the unconscious dimension of our relationships is shown to be important. The relationships between staff, between patients, between staff and patients, staff and those who manage them, workforces and the various bodies and organisations that monitor and govern them—these are shown to be the key to the capacity of mental health staff to hold the psychologically vulnerable patient in mind. This includes the capacity to experience disturbance, in order to offer a form of containment that allows the disturbed patient to feel understood, on a deep level. With this level of thoughtfulness built into the system within which they work, those staff who are sensitive and interested in the minds of their patients, and have not developed—or do not want to develop—thick skins and a rigid, task-based mentality, are less likely to leave full-time employment in mental health services, or to need time off for sickness because they are demoralised and burnt-out. This is good for the workforce as a whole, economically, and also because it reduces disruption to teams, and, hence, interruptions to the continuity of patient care.

The NHS has always had to make the most of scarce resources and to be accountable for its use of the public purse. This book shows some of the ways in which psychoanalysis has applied itself, creatively, to this challenge. Establishing this level of understanding is hard, emotionally, but it can also be rewarding. What makes the work more difficult today, as many of the authors show, is that staff feel themselves to be working on a battleground. The war that they find themselves involved in is not just between health and illness, but between the reparative social values at the heart of our public welfare system and a political belief in a competitive, market approach, which is sometimes described as "neoliberal" (Bell, 2013).

Somehow, in the thick of this battle, mental health staff have to keep their patients, and each other, in mind, while resisting the impulse to act out feelings of anger and frustration, or to collude with the pressure to provide a picture that is more virtual than real, or to take flight through sickness, resignation, and early retirement. To combat such impulses, these authors adopt an analytic stance, of being "observing participants" and "reflective practitioners".

Many commentators are expressing concerns about the effects of our move away from "non-marketised social institutions that . . . bind people together in a collective form, providing a structure for containing and managing human destructiveness and creating a context for collective, reparative effort" (Bell, 2014). Links have been made with other forms of change affecting society, notably the environment, as when Clare Gerada speaks of change that is "too much, and too rapid, and too deep . . . destabilising the complex eco-system that is the NHS—leaving us unable to recover, and adapt, and regain the capacity to care for others (or indeed ourselves)."

In her book on climate change (2012), the psychoanalyst Sally Weintrobe describes a way in which society turns a blind eye to the difficult, anxiety-provoking issue of environmental damage, describing it in psychoanalytic terms as a mental health problem of our contemporary society, involving narcissistic defences that enable us to feel powerful and to deny our part in the despoliation of our world. In order to combat this "culture of uncare", she offers some guiding principles that might help us to change and to begin to develop a "framework of care". In such a culture,

> thinking is an inner, psychic, dynamic building project in which we maintain links with care by keeping those we care for near by us in the

internal world of the imagination, close enough to feel touched by them. A main way we break links to care is by spatially rearranging our relationships in the inner world of the mind in order to keep people at a distance. As "distanced others", we do not care as much for them. An internal world with uncare in charge is an internal world in which our relationships have been reengineered spatially in this kind of way. My argument is the culture of uncare works to promote this kind of rearranging which can lead to a distorted inner represen-tation of the external world. (Weintrobe, 2015)

In this view, mental health problems are a matter of social urgency. Mental health services often do an extraordinary job of taking on board the disturbance and distress of patients suffering from mental health problems. They provide a home for conditions of the mind that may be described as psychologically "toxic". They have much to teach society. But they cannot do it all.

A number of policy-makers and social commentators—not least the *Five Year Forward View*—note the link between our increasingly unequal society and escalating rates of psychological ill health. Poverty and deprivation have been found to correlate to suicide rates and mental illness: the charity Mind estimated in April 2016 that almost half of all people with mental health problems had considered taking, or had attempted to take, their own lives due to social factors such as debt and welfare difficulties. And among the young, Sebastian Kraemer, consultant child and adolescent psychiatrist at the Tavistock Clinic, describes frighteningly high rates of anxiety, depression, and self-harm as "the canary in the mine . . . a warning of the danger we all face . . . The poison in the social atmosphere that is hitting teenagers is their unprecedented lack of prospects in education, employment, and housing" (Kraemer, 2016).

We cannot rely on mental health services to do the environmental equivalent of acting as "green lungs" in the face of a psychologically corrosive culture. As a society, we need to know that many of society's problems with violence (towards the self and towards others), abuse, and other destructive ways of relating, are signs of what Kraemer described as a "poison in the social atmosphere" and Weintrobe (2012) a "culture of uncare". Unless society takes heed of these warnings, it is likely that our mental health services will slowly but surely be rele-gated to the role of fire-fighting—a "repressive" form of containment, in place of the transformative potential these authors describe.

Research shows that the effects of psychoanalytic intervention are long-lasting—the "sleeper" effect. The outcomes from providing staff with psychoanalytically informed help for their own mental processes may be difficult to quantify, but that research challenge is equally important. This book shows the effectiveness of applying analytic insight to all levels of mental health provision. Without this form of mental digestion, there is a danger that these services, rather than providing a structure that can communicate, make links, and contain human distress and disturbance, will instead end up in need of yet another master plan, as patients and staff continue to fail, and be failed by, a system claiming fine-seeming results, while turning a blind eye to working reality.

NOTES

1. The identity of this "book" is a mystery. According to Professor Riccardo Steiner, who kindly gave the matter his attention, the paper on "The psychical mechanism of forgetfulness" was not in circulation during these years but was translated by Alix Strachey for the Freud Standard Edition in the 1950s. Professor Steiner suggests, as an alternative, that the reference could be to Freud's famous essay "On transience", which was translated by Strachey and published in the International Journal of Psychoanalysis in 1942.
2. Psychoanalytically, such myths may be regarded as the equivalent of unconscious phantasies in individuals.
3. Rosenfeld (1971) describes, as part of destructive narcissism, an internal structure, like a gang or "Mafia", which dominates the person internally and, for example, attacks any weakness or vulnerability in the person and in others
4. The Care Quality Commission (CQC) is responsible for examining the quality of clinical work in services in the NHS and private sector and has the power, if there are serious concerns, to enforce special measures or even closures.
5. In 2007, ten beds were cut and the hospital had been reduced from three to two units.

6. Beginning with the ground-breaking research studies of Malan (1976) at the Tavistock Clinic, and more recently summarised by Shedler (2010). See also Bravesmith, 2010.

7. The independence and confidentiality of counselling services for staff are supported by DoH guidelines, which emphasise that the counselling relationship depends on complete confidentiality, so that even in exceptional circumstances—that is, "where failure to disclose information may expose the person themselves, a patient, or others, to risk of death or serious harm"—only as much information as is necessary for the purpose must be disclosed, and the counsellor must ensure that those to whom information is disclosed are aware that this is volunteered in confidence, which must be respected.

8. A recent focus for decision-making around "DNR"—"often a violent process with rib fractures and brain injury significant risks"—was the case of Janet Tracey, who died in hospital shortly before the case Nurse A was involved in. The Court's ruling on the case was reported in a *Guardian* article by James Meikle (2014).

REFERENCES

Adlam, J., & Scanlon, C. (Eds.) (2011). Psycho-social perspectives on the dynamics of inclusion and exclusion in groups, organisations, communities. *Psychodynamic Practice*, *17*(3) (Special Issue on psycho-social perspectives on the dynamics of inclusion and exclusion in groups, organisations and communities).

Adlam, J., Aiyegbusi, A., Kleinot, P., Motz, A., & Scanlon, C. (Eds.) (2012). *The Therapeutic Milieu Under Fire: Security and Insecurity in Forensic Mental Health*. London: Jessica Kingsley.

Agazarian, Y. M. (1997). *Systems-Centered Therapy for Groups*. New York: Guilford Press.

Aiyegbusi, A., & Clarke, J. (Eds.) (2008). *Relationships with Offenders: An Introduction to the Psychodynamics of Forensic Mental Health Nursing*. London: Jessica Kingsley.

Aiyegbusi, A., & Kelly, G. (Eds.) (2012). *Professional and Therapeutic Boundaries in Forensic Mental Health*. London: Jessica Kingsley.

Alvarez, A., & Reid, S. (1999). *Autism and Personality. Findings from the Tavistock Autism Workshop*. London: Routledge.

Argyris, C., & Schön, D. A. (1974). *Theory in Practice: Increasing Professional Effectiveness*. San Francisco. CA: Jossey Bass.

Argyris, C., & Schön, D. A. (1978). *Organisational Learning: A Theory of Action Perspective*. Reading, MA: Addison-Wesley.

Armstrong, D. (2005). *Organization in the Mind: Psychoanalysis, Group Relations and Organizational Consultancy*. London: Karnac.

Armstrong, D., & Rustin, M. (2014). *Social Defences Against Anxiety: Explorations in a Paradigm*. London: Karnac.

Balint, E. (1973). The "flash technique": its freedom and its discipline. In: M. Balint & J. S. Norell (Eds.), *Six Minutes for the Patient: Interactions in General Practice Consultations* (pp. 19–32). London: Tavistock.

Balint, M. (1955). The doctor, his patient, and the illness. *Lancet, 26*: 683–688.

Balint, M. (1957). *The Doctor, His Patient and The Illness*. London: Pitman Medical.

Balint, M. (1964). *The Doctor, His Patient and the Illness* (2nd edn). London: Pitman.

Balint, M., & Balint, E. (1961). *Psychotherapeutic Techniques in Medicine*. London: Tavistock.

Balint, M., & Norell, J. S. (1973). *Six Minutes for the Patient: Interactions in General Practice Consultations*. London: Tavistock.

Ballatt, J., & Campling, P. (2011). *Intelligent Kindness: Reforming the Culture of Healthcare*. London: Royal College of Psychiatrists.

Balsam, R. (1996). The pregnant mother and the body image of the daughter. *Journal of the American Psychoanalytic Association, 44(Suppl.)*: 401–427.

Banks, M. (1997). Unconscious factors in the personality of the healer: an exploration through the psychoanalytic encounter. Unpublished MA thesis, University of Hertfordshire.

Banks, M. (2002). The transition from therapist to supervisor. In: C. Driver & E. Martin (Eds.), *Supervising Psychotherapy: Psychoanalytic and Psychodynamic Perspectives* (pp. 23–37). London: Sage.

Bell, D. (1996). Primitive mind of state. *Psychoanalytic Psychotherapy, 10*: 45–57.

Bell, D. (2013). Mental illness and its treatment today. Centre for Health and the Public Interest. www.chpi.org.uk.

Bell, D. (2014). Psychoanalysis in 2025. www.epf-fep.eu/eng/collection/psychoanalysis-in-2025-pre-published-papers.

Beveridge, W. (1942). *Report on Social Insurance and Allied Services*. London: Stationery Office.

Bick, E. (1964). Infant observation in psychoanalytic training. *International Journal of Psychoanalysis, 45*: 558–566.

Bion, W. R. (1957). Differentiation of the psychotic from the non-psychotic personalities. *International Journal of Psychoanalysis, 38*: 266–275. Reprinted in Bion, W. R. (1967) *Second Thoughts: Selected Papers on Psychoanalysis* (pp. 43–64). London: Karnac.

Bion, W. R. (1959). Attacks on linking. *International Journal of Psycho-analysis, 40:* 308–315. Reprinted in: Bion, W. R. (1967). *Second Thoughts: Selected Papers on Psychoanalysis* (pp. 93–109). London: Karnac.

Bion, W. R. (1961). *Experiences in Groups and Other Papers.* London: Karnac.

Bion, W. R. (1962). A theory of thinking. In: *Second Thoughts: Selected Papers on Psychoanalysis* (pp. 110–119). London: Karnac.

Bion, W. R. (1963). *Elements of Psycho-Analysis.* London: Karnac.

Bion, W. R. (1967). *Second Thoughts: Selected Papers on Psychoanalysis.* London: Karnac.

Blumenthal, S., Ruszczynski, S., Richards, R., & Brown, M. (2011). Evaluation of the impact of a consultation in a secure setting. *Criminal Behaviour and Mental Health, 21:* 233–244.

Boston, M. (1980). Psychotherapy with severely deprived children: intro-duction—the Tavistock Workshop. *Journal of Child Psychotherapy, 6*(1): 45–48.

Box, S., Copley, B., Magagna, J., & Moustaki, E. (1981). *Psychotherapy with Families: An Analytic Approach.* London: Routledge.

Bramley, W. (1990). Staff sensitivity groups: a conductor's field experi-ences. *Group Analysis, 23:* 301–316.

Bravesmith, A. (2010). Can we be brief? *British Journal of Psychotherapy, 26:* 274–290.

Britton, J. (2008). How long is enough? Brief treatment models for adoles-cents and young adults. Unpublished conference paper: Scottish Institute of Human Relations.

Britton, R. (1989). The missing link. In: R. Britton, M. Feldman, & E. O'Shaughnessy (Eds.), *The Oedipus Complex Today* (pp. 83–101). London: Karnac.

Burton, J. (2015). *Leading Good Care: The Task, Heart and Art of Managing Social Care.* London: Jessica Kingsley.

Campling, P., Davies, S., & Farquharson, G. (Eds.) (2004). *From Toxic Institutions to Therapeutic Environments: Residential Settings in Mental Health Services.* London: Royal College of Psychiatrists.

Carlyle, J., & Evans, C. (2005). Containing containers: attention to the "innerface" and "outerface" of groups in secure institutions. *Group Analysis, 38*(3): 395–408.

Carson, J., & Dennison, P. (2008). The role of groupwork in tackling organ-isational burnout: two contrasting perspectives. *Groupwork, 18*(2): 18–25.

Casement, P. (1985). *Learning from the Patient.* London: Routledge.

Casement, P. (2002). *Learning from our Mistakes: Beyond Dogma in Psycho-analysis and Psychotherapy.* Harmondsworth: Brunner-Routledge.

Castle, D., McGrath, J., & Kulkarni, J. (2000). *Women and Schizophrenia*. Cambridge: Cambridge University Press.

Chiesa, M. (1993). At the border between institutionalization and community psychiatry: psychodynamic observations of a hospital admission ward. *Free Associations, 4:* 241–263.

Chiesa, M., Fonagy, P., & Holmes, J. (2006). Six-year follow-up of three treatment programs to personality disorder. *Journal of Personality Disorders, 20*(5): 493–509.

Chodorow, N. (1978). *The Reproduction of Mothering: Psychoanalysis and the Sociology of Gender*. Berkeley, CA: University of California Press.

Coltart, N. (1992). The practice of psychoanalysis and Buddhism. In: *Slouching Towards Bethlehem and Further Psychoanalytic Explorations* (pp. 164–175). London: Free Association Books.

Connors, D. D. (1988). A continuum of researcher–participant relationships: an analysis and critique. *Advances in Nursing Science, 10*(4): 12–35.

Cooper, A., & Lousada, J. (2005). *Borderline Welfare: Feeling and Fear of Feeling in Modern Welfare*. London: Karnac.

Copley, B., & Forryan, B. (1997). *Therapeutic Work with Children and Young People*. London: Cassell.

Cornes, M., Manthorpe, J., Hennessey, C., Anderson, S., Clark, M., & Scanlon, C. (2014). Not just a talking shop: practitioner perspectives on how communities of practice work to improve outcomes for people experiencing multiple exclusion homelessness. *Journal of Interprofessional Care, 28*(6): 541–546.

Cotton, E. (2016). Start where you are. British Psychoanalytic Council publication. *New Associations, 20*.

Craib, I. (1994). *The Importance of Disappointment*. London: Routledge.

Crichton Miller, H. (1920). *Functional Nerve Disease: An Epitome of War Experience for the Practitioner*. London: H. Frowde; Hodder & Stoughton.

Cummins, A. M. (2002). 'The road to hell is paved with good intentions': quality assurance as a social defence against anxiety. *Organisational and Social Dynamics, 2*(1): 99–119.

Cutler, I. (2005). *Cynicism from Diogenes to Dilbert*. London: McFarland.

Dartington, A. (1994). Where angels fear to tread. In: A. Obholzer & V. Zagier Roberts (Eds.), *The Unconscious at Work: Individual and Organizational Stress in the Human Services* (pp. 101–109). London: Routledge.

Dartington, T. (1986). *The Limits of Altruism: Elderly Mentally Infirm People as a Test Case for Collaboration*. London: King Edward's Hospital Fund for London.

Dartington, T. (2010). *Managing Vulnerability: The Underlying Dynamics of Systems of Care*. London: Karnac.

Davids, M. F. (2011). *Internal Racism: A Psychoanalytic Approach to Race and Difference*. Basingstoke: Palgrave-Macmillan.

Department for Communities and Local Government (2010). *Meeting the Psychological and Emotional Needs of Homeless People: Non-statutory Guidance on Dealing with Complex Psychological and Emotional Needs*. HMSO: Department for Communities and Local Government.

Department for Educational and Skills/Department of Health (2006). *Report on the Implementation of Standard 9 of the National Service Framework for Children, Young People and Maternity Services. Annex: Models of Good Practice*. London: HMSO.

Department of Health (2002). *Women's Mental Health: Into the Mainstream. Strategic Development of Mental Health Care for Women*. London: HMSO.

Department of Health (2013). *Integrated Care and Support: Our Shared Commitment*. London: HMSO.

Department of Health, NHS England (2004). *National Service Framework*. London: HMSO.

Department of Health, NHS England (2015). *Future in Mind—Promoting, Protecting and Improving our Children and Young People's Mental Health and Wellbeing*. London: HMSO.

Dicks, H. V. (1970). *Fifty Years of the Tavistock Clinic*. London: Routledge & Kegan Paul.

Drennan, G., Casado, S., & Minchin, L. (2014). Dilemmas and ethical decision making: reflective practice in community settings. In: Z. Ashmore & R. Shuker (Eds.), *Forensic Practice in the Community* (pp. 35–47). London: Routledge.

Dwight Culler, A. (1961). *Poetry and Criticism of Matthew Arnold*. Boston: Houghton Mifflin.

Dwyer, D. (1995). Response to the victims of domestic violence: analysis and implications of the British experience. *Crime & Delinquency, 41*: 527–540.

Eckstein, R., & Wallerstein, R. S. (1958). *The Teaching and Learning of Psychotherapy*. New York: Basic Books.

Emanuel, L. (2002). Deprivation x 3: the contribution of organisational dynamics to the "triple deprivation" of looked after children. *Journal of Child Psychotherapy, 28*(2): 163–177.

Enckell, H. (2002). *Metaphor and the Psychodynamic Functions of the Mind*. Kuopio: Kuopio University Press.

Evans, M. (2014). "I'm beyond caring": a response to the Francis Report. *Psychoanalytic Psychotherapy, 28*: 193–210.

Fabricius, J. (1995). Psychoanalytic understanding and nursing: a supervisory workshop with nurse tutors. *Psychoanalytic Psychotherapy, 9*: 17–29.

Fagin, L. (2001). Therapeutic and counter-therapeutic factors in acute ward settings. *Psychoanalytic Psychotherapy, 15*: 99–120.

Fenichel, O. (1946). *The Psychological Theory of Neurosis.* London: Routledge & Kegan Paul.

Fonagy, P., & Bateman, A. (2006). *Mentalized Based Treatment for Borderline Personality Disorder.* Oxford: Oxford University Press.

Fonagy, P., & Lemma, A. (2012). Does psychoanalysis have a valuable place in modern mental health services? Yes. *British Medical Journal, 344*: e1211.

Fonagy, P., & Target, M. (1996). Playing with reality: 1. Theory of mind and the normal development of psychic reality. *International Journal of Psychoanalysis, 77*: 217–233.

Fonagy, P., Gergely, G., Jurist, E. L., & Target, M. (2003). The social biofeedback theory of affect mirroring: the development of emotional self-awareness and self-control. In: *Affect Regulation, Mentalization, and the Development of the Self* (pp. 145–202). London: Karnac.

Fonagy, P., Rost, F., Carlyle, J., McPherson, S., Thomas, R., Fearon, P., Goldberg, D., & Taylor, D. (2015). Pragmatic randomized controlled trial of long-term psychoanalytic psychotherapy for treatment-resistant depression: the Tavistock Adult Depression Study (TADS). *World Psychiatry, 14*: 312–321.

Foulkes, S. H. (1973). The group as matrix of the individual's mental life. In: L. R. Wolberg & E. K. Schwartz (Eds.), *Group Therapy* (pp. 211–220). New York: Intercontinental Medical Books.

Foulkes, S. H., & Anthony, E. J. (1965). *Group Psychotherapy: The Psychoanalytic Approach* (Maresfield Library). London: Karnac.

Francis, R. (2010). [First report] *The Independent Inquiry into Care Provided by Mid-Staffordshire NHS Foundation Trust, January 2005–March 2009.* London: HMSO.

Francis, R. (2013). *The Mid Staffordshire NHS Foundation Trust Public Inquiry Chaired by Robert Francis QC HC 947. Report of the Mid Staffordshire NHS Foundation Trust Public Inquiry.* London: HMSO.

French, R. (2001). "Negative capability": managing the confusing uncertainties of change. *Journal of Organizational Change Management, 14*(5): 480–492.

Freud, S. (1909b). *Analysis of a Phobia in a Five-Year-Old Boy. S. E., 10*: 1–150. London: Hogarth.

Freud, S. (1910d). The future prospects of psycho-analytic therapy. *S. E., 11*: 139–152. London: Hogarth.

Freud, S. (1919a). Lines of advance in psycho-analytic therapy. *S. E., 17:* 159–168. London: Hogarth.

Freud, S. (1920g). *Beyond the Pleasure Principle. S. E., 18:* 7–64. London: Hogarth.

Freud, S. (1923b). *The Ego and the Id. S. E., 19:* 3–66. London: Hogarth.

Freud, S. (1926d). *Inhibitions, Symptoms and Anxiety. S. E., 20:* 77–175. London: Hogarth.

Freud, S. (1937c). Analysis terminable and interminable. *S. E., 23:* 209–254. London: Hogarth.

Gabbard, G. O., & Wilkinson, S. (1994). *Management of Counter-transference with Borderline Patients.* Washington, DC: American Psychiatric Press.

Garelick, A. I. (2012). Doctors' health: stigma and the professional discomfort in seeking help. *The Psychiatrist, 36*(3): 81–84.

Garner, J. (2014). Some thoughts and responses to The Francis Report. *Psychoanalytic Psychotherapy, 28:* 211–219.

Gawande, A. (2014). *Being Mortal: Medicine and What Matters in the End.* London: Profile Books.

Gay, P. (1988). *Freud: A Life for Our Time.* London: Dent.

Gerada, C. (2014). Something is profoundly wrong with the NHS today. *BMJ,* 16 June 2014.

Gilligan, J. (1996). *Violence: Reflections on our Deadliest Epidemic.* London: Jessica Kingsley.

Goldberg, D., & Taylor, D. (2015). Pragmatic randomized controlled trial of long-term psychoanalytic psychotherapy for treatment-resistant depression: the Tavistock Adult Depression Study (TADS). *World Psychiatry, 14*(3): 312–321.

Gordon, J., & Kirtchuk, G. (Eds.) (2008). *Psychic Assaults and Frightened Clinicians: Counter-transference in Forensic Settings.* London: Karnac.

Griffiths, P., & Hinshelwood, R. D. (2001). Enquiring into a culture of enquiry. In: L. Day & P. Pringle (Eds.), *Reflective Enquiry into Therapeutic Institutions* (pp. 29–44). London: Karnac.

Grotstein, J. S. (1984). A proposed revision of the psychoanalytic concept of primitive mental states, Part II: the borderline syndrome—section 2: the phenomenology of the borderline syndrome. *Contemporary Psychoanalysis, 20:* 77–119.

Haigh, R. (2000). Support systems. 2. Staff sensitivity groups. *Advances in Psychiatric Treatment, 6:* 312–319.

Halton, W. (1995). Institutional stress on providers in health and education. *Psychodynamic Counselling, 1*(2): 187–198.

Harris Williams, M. (Ed.) (2011). The Tavistock Model: Papers on Child Development and Psychoanalytic Training by Martha Harris and

Esther Bick. Vol. 1 of *The Collected Papers of Martha Harris and Esther Harris*. London: Karnac.

Hartley, P., & Kennard, D. (Eds.) (2009). *Staff Support Groups in the Helping Professions: Principles and Pitfalls*. London: Routledge.

Herman, J. (1992). *Trauma and Recovery: From Domestic Violence to Political Terror*. London: Pandora.

Hinshelwood, R. D. (1989). *A Dictionary of Kleinian Thought*. London: Free Association Books.

Hinshelwood, R. D. (1995). Psychoanalysis in Britain: points of cultural access, 1893–1918. *International Journal of Psychoanalysis, 76:* 135–151.

Hinshelwood, R. D., & Manning, N. P. (1979). *Therapeutic Communities: Reflections and Progress*. London: Routledge.

Hinshelwood, R. D., & Skogstad, W. (1998). The hospital in the mind: the setting and the internal world. In-patient psychotherapy at the Cassel Hospital. In: J. Pestalozzi (Ed.), *Psychoanalytic Psychotherapy in Institutional Settings* (pp. 59–73). London: Karnac.

Hinshelwood, R. D., & Skogstad, W. (2000). *Observing Organisations: Anxiety, Defence and Culture in Health Care*. London: Routledge.

Hobson, P. (2002). *The Cradle of Thought*. London: Pan Macmillan.

Hoggett, P. (2010). Perverse social structures. *Journal of Psychosocial Studies*, 4(1): 57–64.

Holtzman, D., & Kulish, N. (2000). The femininization of the female oedipal complex, Part I. *Journal of the American Psychoanaytic Association, 48:* 1413–1437.

Holtzman, D., & Kulish, N. (2003). The femininization of the female oedipal complex, Part II: Aggression reconsidered. *Journal of the American Psychoanalytic Association, 51:* 1127–1151.

Honig, B. (1996). Difference, dilemmas and the politics of home. In: S. Benhabib (Ed.), *Democracy and Difference: Contesting the Boundaries of the Political* (pp. 257–277). Princeton: Princeton University Press.

Hopper, E. (2003). *Traumatic Experience in the Unconscious Life of Groups: The Fourth Basic Assumption: Incohesion: Aggregation/Massification or (ba) I:A/M*. London: Jessica Kingsley.

Hopper, E. (2011). *Trauma in Organisations*. London: Karnac.

Hume, F., & Kleeberg, B. (2004). Playing a poor hand well: succumbing to or triumphing over developmental adversity: a study of adults sexually abused in care. In: S. Levy & A. Lemma (Eds.), *The Perversion of Loss: Psychoanalytic Perspectives on Trauma* (pp. 71–86). London: Whurr.

Illiffe, S. (2008). *From General Practice to Primary Care: the Industrialisation of Family Medicine*. Oxford: Oxford University Press.

Independent Mental Health Taskforce (2016). Report to the NHS in England. www.england.nhs.uk/mentalhealth/taskforce

James, C. (1994). Holding and containing in the group and in society. In: D. Brown & L. Zinkin (Eds.), *The Psyche and the Social World*. London: Routledge.

Jameson, F. (1991). *Postmodernism or The Cultural Logic of Late Capitalism*. London: Verso.

Jaques, E. (1955). Social systems as a defence against persecutory and depressive anxiety. In: M. Klein, P. Heimann, & R. Money-Kyrle (Eds.), *New Directions in Psycho-Analysis* (pp. 478–498). New York: Basic Books.

Johns Hopkins Newsroom (2013). PTSD symptoms common among ICU survivors [press release: 26 February 2013]. Birmingham, AL: Newswise.

Johnson, R., & Haigh, R. (2010). Social psychiatry and social policy for the 21st century—new concepts for new needs: the "psychologically-informed environment". *Mental Health and Social Inclusion, 14*(4): 30–35.

Johnson, R., & Haigh, R. (2011). Social psychiatry and social policy for the 21st century: new concepts for new needs—the "Enabling Environments" initiative. *Mental Health and Social Inclusion, 15*(1): 17–26.

Johnston, J. (2017). *Learning from the Cradle to the Grave: the Psychotherapeutic Development of Doctors from the Beginning to the End of their Career in Medicine and Psychiatry*. Royal College of Psychiatrists Occasional Paper 102.

Jones, M. (1968). *Social Psychiatry in Practice: The Idea of the Therapeutic Community*. Harmondsworth: Penguin.

Joseph, B. (1985). Transference: the total situation. *International Journal of Psychoanalysis, 66:* 447–454.

Judt, T. (2010). *Ill Fares the Land*. Harmondsworth: Penguin.

Kanas, N. (1986). Support groups for mental health staff. *International Journal of Group Psychotherapy, 36:* 279–296.

Karpman, S. (1968). Fairy tales and script drama analysis. *Transactional Analysis Bulletin, 7*(26): 39–43.

Keats, J. (1970)[1817]. Letter to his brothers, 21 December. In: R. Gittings (Ed.), *The Letters of John Keats: a Selection* (pp. 41–43). Oxford: Oxford University Press.

Keenan, A., Smyth, P., & Thomaidis-Zades, K. (2013). Complexity factors in the presentation of children and adolescents in child psychotherapy. *Association of Child Psychotherapists Bulletin, 247:* 7–13.

Kennedy, E. (2015). Developing interventions in child and adolescent mental health services: do we really know what works for whom? *Clinical Child Psychology and Psychiatry, 20*(4): 529–531.

Kennedy, R. (2002). A history of the closure threat to the Cassel Hospital. In: *Psychoanalysis, History and Subjectivity* (pp. 31–48). London: Routledge.

Khaleelee, O., & Miller, E. (1985). Beyond the small group: society as an intelligible field of study. In: M. Pines (Ed.), *Bion and Group Psychotherapy* (pp. 354–385). London: Routledge & Kegan Paul.

Kipling, R. (1940). *The Definitive Edition of the Verse of Rudyard Kipling (1865–1936)*. London: Hodder & Stoughton.

Klein, M. (1929). Infantile anxiety situations reflected in a work of art and in the creative impulse. In: *Love, Guilt and Reparation and Other Works, 1921–1945* (pp. 210–218). London: Hogarth.

Klein, M. (1933). The early development of conscience in the child. In: *Love, Guilt and Reparation and Other Works, 1921–1945* (pp. 248–257). London: Hogarth.

Klein, M. (1940). Mourning and its relation to manic-depressive states. *International Journal of Psychoanalysis, 21:* 125–153.

Klein, M. (1946). Notes on some schizoid mechanisms. *International Journal of Psychoanalysis, 27:* 1–24.

Kraemer, S. (2016). Letter to the Editor. *Observer* Comment, 22 May.

Kulish, N. (2002). Female sexuality. *Psychoanalytic Study of the Child, 57:* 151–176.

Kulish, N., & Holtzman, D. (2003). Counter-transference and the female triangular situation. *International Journal of Psychoanalysis, 84:* 563–577.

Lakoff, G., & Johnson, M. (1980). *Metaphors We Live By*. Chicago, IL: University of Chicago Press.

Lakoff, G., & Johnson, M. (1999). *Philosophy in the Flesh: The Embodied Mind and its Challenge to Western Thought*. New York: Basic Books.

Lees, A., & Meyer, E. (2011). Theoretically speaking: use of communities of practice framework to describe and evaluate interprofessional education. *Journal of Interprofessional Care, 25:* 84–90.

Lerner, H. F. (1980). Internal prohibitions against female anger. *American Journal of Psychoanalysis, 40:* 137–147.

Lévi-Strauss, C. (1978). "Primitive" thinking and the "civilised" mind. In: *Myth and Meaning: the Massey Lectures*. London: Routledge & Kegan Paul.

Lodge, G. (2012). How did we let it come to this? A plea for the principle of continuity of care. *The Psychiatrist Online, 36:* 361–363.

Loyal, S., & Quilley, S. (2004). *The Sociology of Norbert Elias*. Cambridge: Cambridge University Press.

Luft, J. (1982). *The Johari Window: A Graphic Model of Awareness in Interpersonal Relations*. San Francisco, CA: NTL Laboratories.

Maher, M. J. (2009). Authority and control: working with staff croups in children's homes. In: P. Hartley & D. Kennard (Eds.), *Staff Support Groups in the Helping Professions: Principles and Pitfalls* (pp. 122–134). London: Routledge.

Main, T. F. (1967). Knowledge, learning and freedom from thought. In: L. Day & P. Pringle (Eds.), *Reflective Enquiry into Therapeutic Institutions* (pp. 1–22). London: Karnac, 2001.

Main, T. F. (1989a). The concept of the therapeutic community: variations and vicissitudes. In: *The Ailment and Other Psychoanalytic Essays* (pp. 124–142). London: Free Association Books.

Main, T. F. (1989b). *The Ailment and Other Psychoanalytic Essays*. London: Free Association Books.

Malan, D. (1976). *The Frontier of Brief Psychotherapy: An Example of Convergence of Research and Clinical Practice*. London: Plenum Press.

Marsh, H. (2014). *Do No Harm*. London: Orion.

McCarron, E. (2015). *The Future of General Practice—GP Career Motivations and Workforce Crisis. A GP Executive Committee Survey*. London: British Medical Association.

McDougall, V., Luckett, K., & Jones, M. (2007). Women's experience of psychosis. In: R. Velleman, E. Davis, G. Smith, & M. Drage (Eds.), *Changing Outcomes in Psychosis* (pp. 117–134). Oxford: Wiley-Blackwell.

McQueen, D. (2009). Association for Psychoanalytic Psychotherapy in the NHS, The Anna Freud Centre, British Psychoanalytic Council, The Tavistock and Portman NHS Foundation Trust. *Response to the NICE Clinical Guideline on Depression*. London: British Psychoanalytic Council.

McQueen, D., & St John Smith, P. (2015). NICE recommendations for psychotherapy in depression: of limited clinical utility. *Psychiatrike*, 26(3): 188–197.

Meikle, J. (2014). Hospital violated patient's right with 'Do Not Resuscitate' order, Court rules. *Guardian*, 17 June.

Meltzer, D. (1978). Container and contained: the prototype of learning. In: *The Kleinian Development Part III: The Clinical Significance of the Work of Bion* (pp. 46–53). Strathtay, Perthshire: Clunie Press.

Menzies, A. C. (1960). *Frank Twyman: 1876–1959. Biographical Memoirs of the Royal Society*. London: Royal Society.

Menzies Lyth, I. (1988a[1959a]). *Containing Anxiety in Institutions: Selected Essays*. London: Free Association Books.

Menzies Lyth, I. (1988b[1959b]). The functioning of social systems as a defence against anxiety. *Human Relations, 13*: 95–121. Reprinted in: *Containing Anxiety in Institutions: Selected Papers (Volume 1)*. London: Free Association Books.

Menzies Lyth, I. (1989). *The Dynamics of the Social: Selected Essays*. London: Free Association Books.

Midgley, N., & Kennedy, E. (2011). Psychodynamic psychotherapy for children and adolescents: a critical review of the evidence base. *Journal of Child Psychotherapy, 37*: 232–257.

Midgley, N., Anderson, J., Grainger, E., Nesic-Vuckovic, T., & Urwin, C. (2009). *Child Psychotherapy and Research: New Approaches, Emergent Findings*. Hove: Routledge.

Midgley, N., Cregeen, S., Hughes, C., & Rustin, M. (2013). Psychodynamic psychotherapy as treatment for depression in adolescence. *Child and Adolescent Psychiatry Clinics of North America, 22*: 67–82.

Miller, L. (1992). The relation of infant observation to clinical practice in an under-fives counselling service. *Journal of Child Psychotherapy, 18*: 19–32.

Miller, L., Rustin, M., Rustin, M., & Shuttleworth, J. (1989). *Closely Observed Infants*. London: Duckworth.

Miller, M. (1975). Transference and counter-transference in action—an ABC of three organisational levels: a case study. Presentation to St Bartholomew's Hospital. Department of Psychiatry/City of London Social Services/Hackney Social Services, 4 November.

Mills, T., & Smith, M. (2015). Metabolizing difficult doctor–patient relationships: reflections on a Balint group for higher trainees. *British Journal of Psychotherapy, 31*: 390–400.

Morgan, D. (2014). Personal communication.

Moustaki, E. (1981). Glossary: a discussion and application of terms. In: S. Box, B. Copley, J. Magagna, & E. Moustaki (Eds.), *Psychotherapy with Families* (pp. 127–133). London: Routledge.

Music, G. (2009). Neglecting neglect: some thoughts about children who have lacked good input, and are "undrawn" and "unenjoyed". *Psychoanalytic Psychotherapy, 35*(2): 142–156.

Navia, L. (2005). *Diogenes the Cynic*. New York: Humanity Books.

NHS England, Care Quality Commission, Health Education England, Monitor, Public Health England, Trust Development Authority, & NICE (2014). *The Five Year Forward View*.

Nietzsche, F. (1886). *Beyond Good and Evil*, W. Kaufmann (Trans.). New York: Random House, 1966.

Norton, K., & Dolan, B. (1995). Acting out and the institutional response. *Journal of Forensic Psychiatry*, 6(2): 317–333.

Novakovic, A. (2002). Work with psychotic patients in a rehabilitation unit: a short term staff support group with a nursing team. *Group Analysis*, 35(4): 560–573.

Obholzer, A. (1994). Managing social anxieties in public sector organizations. In: A. Obholzer & V. Roberts (Eds.), *The Unconscious at Work: Individual and Organizational Stress in the Human Services* (pp. 169–178). London: Routledge.

Obholzer, A., & Roberts, V. Z. (Eds.) (1994). *The Unconscious at Work: Individual and Organizational Stress in the Human Services*. London: Routledge.

O'Connor, S. (1998). An analytic approach in a psychiatric intensive care unit. *Psychoanalytic Psychotherapy*, 12: 3–15.

O'Connor, S. (1999). Understanding violent behaviour within the boundaries of a locked ward. *Psychoanalytic Psychotherapy*, 13: 3–17.

Ormrod, S., Ferlie, E., Warren, F., & Norton, K. (2007). The appropriation of new organizational forms within networks of practice: founder and founder-related ideological power. *Human Relations*, 60(5): 745–767.

Padel, R. (2005). *Tigers in Red Weather*. London: Little, Brown.

Payne, S. (1995). The rationing of psychiatric beds: changing trends in sex-ratios in admission to psychiatric hospital. *Health and Social Care in the Community*, 3: 289–300.

Pietroni, M., & Vaspe, A. (2000). *Understanding Counselling in Primary Care: Voices from the Inner City*. London: Churchill Livingstone.

Pietroni, P. (2015). Compassion in Health Care. Keynote Lecture, International Institute for the Study of Compassion, launch conference, 6 October.

Pollitt, C., & Bouckaert, G. (2004). *Public Management Reform: a Comparative Analysis*. Oxford: Oxford University Press.

Rapoport, R. N. (1960). *Community as Doctor*. London: Tavistock.

Redl, F. (1959). The concept of a "therapeutic milieu". *American Journal of Orthopsychiatry*, 29(4): 721–736.

Reiss, D., & Kirtchuk, G. (2009). Interpersonal dynamics and multidisciplinary team work. *Advances in Psychiatric Treatment*, 15: 462–469.

Rhode, M., & Klauber, T. (2004). *The Many Faces of Asperger's Syndrome*. London: Karnac.

Rifkind, G. (1995). Containing the containers: the staff consultation group. *Group Analysis*, 28: 209–222.

Roberts, V. Z. (1994a). The self-assigned impossible task. In: A. Obholzer & V. Roberts (Eds.), *The Unconscious at Work: Individual and Organizational Stress in the Human Services* (pp. 110–118). London: Routledge.

Roberts, V. Z. (1994b). Till death us do part: caring and uncaring in work with the elderly. In: A. Obholzer & V. Z. Roberts (Eds.), *The Unconscious at Work: Individual and Organizational Stress in the Human Services* (pp. 75–83). London: Routledge.

Rosenfeld, H. (1952). Notes on the analysis of a super-ego conflict in an acute catatonic schizophrenic. *International Journal of Psychoanalysis, 33*: 111–131.

Rosenfeld, H. A. (1965). An investigation into the need of neurotic and psychotic patients to act out during analysis. In: *Psychotic States* (pp. 200–216). London: Hogarth.

Rosenfeld, H. A. (1971). A clinical approach to the psychoanalytic theory of the life and death instincts: an investigation into the aggressive aspects of narcissism. *International Journal of Psychoanalysis, 52*: 169–178.

Roth, P., & Fonagy, P. (1996). *What Works for Whom?* New York: Guilford Press.

Rustin, M. (1999). Multiple families in mind. *Clinical Child Psychology and Psychiatry, 4*: 51–62.

Rustin, M. (2008). Work discussion: some historical and theoretical observations. In: M. Rustin & J. Bradley (Eds.), *Work Discussion: Learning from Reflective Practice in Work with Children and Families* (pp. 3–21). London: Karnac.

Ryle, G. (1949). *The Concept of Mind*. London: Hutchinson.

Salzberger-Wittenberg, I., Henry, G., & Osborne, E. (1983). *The Emotional Experience of Learning and Teaching*. London: Karnac.

Sanders, K. (1984). *A Matter of Interest: Clinical Notes of a Psycho-analyst in General Practice*. Strathtay, Perthshire: Clunie Press.

Scanlon, C. (2002). Group supervision of individual cases in the training of psychodynamic practitioners: towards a group-analytic model? *British Journal of Psychotherapy, 19*(2): 219–235.

Scanlon, C. (2012). The traumatised organisation-in-the-mind: creating and maintaining spaces for difficult conversations in difficult places. In: J. Adlam, A. Aiyegbusi, P. Kleinot, A. Motz & C. Scanlon (Eds.), *The Therapeutic Milieu Under Fire: Security and Insecurity in Forensic Mental Health* (pp. 212–228). London: Jessica Kingsley.

Scanlon, C., & Adlam, J. (2008). Refusal, social exclusion and the cycle of rejection: a *cynical* analysis? *Critical Social Policy, 28*(4): 529–549.

Scanlon, C., & Adlam, J. (2011a). Who watches the watchers? Observing the dangerous liaisons between forensic patients and their carers in the perverse panopticon. *Organisational and Social Dynamics, 11*(2): 175–195.

Scanlon, C., & Adlam, J. (2011b). Disorganised responses to refusal and spoiling in traumatised organisations. In: E. Hopper (Ed.), *Trauma and Organisations* (pp. 151–172). London: Karnac.

Scanlon, C., & Adlam, J. (2011c). "Defacing the currency": a group-analytic · appreciation of homelessness, dangerousness, disorder and other inarticulate speech of the heart? *Group Analysis, 44*(2): 131–148.

Scanlon, C., & Adlam, J. (2012). "Dangerous liaisons": close encounters of the un-boundaried kind. In: A. Aiyegbusi & G. Kelly (Eds.), *Professional and Therapeutic Boundaries in Forensic Mental Health Practice* (pp. 240–252). London: Jessica Kingsley.

Scanlon, C., & Weir, W. S. (1997). Learning from practice? Mental health nurses' perceptions and experiences of clinical supervision. *Journal of Advanced Nursing, 26*: 295–303.

Schön, D. A. (1971). *Beyond the Stable State*. New York: Basic Books.

Schön, D. A. (1983). *The Reflective Practitioner: How Professionals Think in Action*. New York: Basic Books.

Schön, D. A. (1987). *Educating the Reflective Practitioner: Toward a New Design for Teaching and Learning in the Professions*. San Francisco, CA: Jossey-Bass.

Senge, P. M. (1990). *The Fifth Discipline: The Art and Practice of the Learning Organisation*. London: Doubleday.

Sharpe, E. F. (1940). *Dream Analysis: a Practical Book for Psycho-Analysts*. London: Hogarth.

Shedler, J. (2010). The efficacy of psychodynamic psychotherapy. *American Psychologist, 65*(2): 98–109.

Shine, J. (2010). Working with offence paralleling in a therapeutic community setting. In: M. Daffern, L. Jones & J. Shine (Eds.), *Offence Paralleling Behaviour: A Case Formulation Approach to Offender Management and Intervention*. Chichester: Wiley- Blackwell.

Shuttleworth, A. (1999). Finding new clinical pathways in the changing world of district child psychotherapy. *Journal of Child Psychotherapy, 25*(1): 29–50.

Simpson, I. (2010). Containing the uncontainable: a role for staff support groups. In: J. Radcliffe, K. Hajek, J. Carson & O. Manor (Eds.), *Psychological Groupwork with Acute Psychiatric Inpatients* (pp. 87–105). London: Whiting & Birch.

Simpson, I. (2016). Containing anxiety in social care systems and neo-liberal management dogma. In: J. Lees (Ed.), *The Future of Psychological Therapy: From Managed Care to Transformational Practice* (pp. 51–68). London: Routledge.

Skogstad, W. (2001). Internal and external reality: enquiring into their interplay in an inpatient setting. In: L. Day & P. Pringle (Eds.), *Reflective Enquiry into Therapeutic Institutions* (pp. 45–65). London: Karnac.

Skogstad, W. (2006) Action and thought: inpatient treatment of severe personality disorders within a psychotherapeutic milieu. In: C. Newrith, C. Meux & P. Taylor (Eds.), *Personality Disorder and Serious Offending* (pp. 161–169). London: Hodder-Arnold.

Skogstad, W. (2012). Does the Cassel have a future? Some facts and thoughts on an historical psychoanalytic institution. *Bulletin of the British Psychoanalytical Society, 48*(1): 24–30.

Skogstad, W. (2014). The Cassel does have a future! Further facts and thoughts on an historical psychoanalytic institution. *Bulletin of the British Psychoanalytical Society, 50*(1): 47–48.

Smith, P. (1992). *The Emotional Labour of Nursing.* Basingstoke: Macmillan.

Soanes, C. (Ed.) (1998). *English Oxford Dictionary.* Oxford: Oxford University Press.

Soubhi, H., Bayliss, E., Fortin, M., Hudon, C., Van den Acker, M., Thivierge, R., Posel, N., & Fleiszer, D. (2010). Learning and caring in communities of practice: using relationships and collective learning to improve primary care for patients with multimorbidity. *Annals of Family Medicine, 8*(2): 170–177.

Stacey, R. (2003). *Complexity and Group Process: A Radically Social Understanding of Individuals.* London: Routledge.

Stanton, A. H., & Schwartz, M. S. (1954). *The Mental Hospital.* New York: Basic Books.

Stokes, J. (2015). Defences against anxiety in the law. In: D. Armstrong & M. Rustin (Eds.), *Social Defences Against Anxiety, Explorations of a Paradigm* (pp. 222–235). London: Karnac.

Symington, J., & Symington, N. (1996). *The Clinical Thinking of Wilfrid Bion.* London: Routledge.

Taylor, D., Carlyle, J., McPherson, S., Rost, F., Thomas, R., & Fonagy, P. (2012). Tavistock Adult Depression Study (TADS). A randomised controlled trial of psychoanalytic psychotherapy for treatment-resistant/treatment-refractory forms of depression. *Bio Med Central (BMC) Psychiatry, 12*: Article 60.

Taylor, F. W. (1911). *The Principles of Scientific Management.* New York: Harper.

Thorndycraft, B., & McCabe, J. (2008). The challenge of working with staff groups in the caring professions: the importance of the "team development and reflective practice group". *British Journal of Psychotherapy*, 24(2): 167–183.

Tillich, P. (1952). *The Courage to Be*. New Haven, CT: Yale University Press.

Timimi, S. (2015). Children and young people's improving access to psychological therapies: inspiring innovation or more of the same? *British Journal of Psychiatry Bulletin, 39*: 57–60.

Trevarthen, C. (1998). The concept and foundations of infant intersubjectivity. In: S. Braten (Ed.), *Intersubjective Communication and Emotion in Early Ontogeny* (pp. 15–46). Cambridge: Cambridge University Press.

Trowell, J., Joffe, I., Campbell, J., Clemente, C., Almqwist, F., Soinen, M., Koskenranta-Aalto, U., Weintraub, S., Kolaitis, G., Tomaras, V., Anastasopoulos, D., Grayson, K., Barnes, J., & Tsiantis, J. (2007). Childhood depression: a place for psychotherapy—an outcome study comparing individual psychodynamic psychotherapy and family therapy. *European Child and Adolescent Psychiatry, 16*: 157–167.

Turquet, P. (1975). Threats to identity in the large group. In: L. Kreeger (Ed.), *The Large Group, Dynamics and Therapy* (pp. 87–144). London: Constable.

Van der Kolk, B. (2014). *The Body Keeps the Score: Mind, Brain and Body in the Transformation of Trauma*. London: Allen Lane.

Vygotsky, L. (1978). *Mind in Society: Development of Higher Psychological Processes*. Cambridge, MA: Harvard University Press.

Waddell, M. (2002[1998]). *Inside Lives*. London: Karnac.

Weintrobe, S. (2012). *Engaging with Climate Change: Psychoanalytic and Interdisciplinary Perspectives*. Hove: Routledge.

Weintrobe, S. (2015). The new imagination in the culture of uncare. Keynote address: Sheffield School of Architecture International Conference. www.sallyweintrobe.com.

Welldon, E. V. (1988). *Mother, Madonna, Whore. The Idealization and Denigration of Motherhood*. London: Karnac.

Wenger, E. (1998). *Communities of Practice*. Cambridge. Cambridge University Press.

White, S. (2013). *An Introduction to the Psychodynamics of Workplace Bullying*. London: Karnac.

Whiteley, J. S. (1986). Sociotherapy and psychotherapy in the treatment of personality disorder: a discussion paper. *Journal of the Royal Society of Medicine, 79*: 721–725.

Wiener, J., & Sher, M. (1998). *Counselling and Psychotherapy in Primary Health Care: a Psychodynamic Approach*. London: Macmillan.

Wilke, G. (2005). Beyond Balint: a group-analysis support model for traumatised doctors. *Group Analysis, 38*: 265–280.

Wilke, G., Freeman, S., & Hilton, S. (2000). *How to Be a Good Enough GP: Surviving and Thriving in the New Primary Care Organisations.* London: Taylor & Francis.

Wilkinson, R., & Pickett, K. (2009). *The Spirit Level: Why More Equal Societies Almost Always Do Better.* London: Allen Lane.

Willis Commission on Nursing Education (2012). *Quality with Compassion: The Future of Nursing Education.* London: Royal College of Nursing.

Winnicott, D. W. (1953). Transitional objects and transitional phenomena. *International Journal of Psychoanalysis, 34*: 89–97.

Winnicott, D. W. (1960). The theory of the parent–infant relationship. *International Journal of Psychoanalysis, 41*: 585–595.

Winnicott, D. W (1990). *The Maturational Processes and the Facilitating Environment: Studies in the Theory of Emotional Development.* London: Maresfield Library.

INDEX

259

270   INDEX

Printed in the United States
by Baker & Taylor Publisher Services